Radiation Brain Moms
and Citizen Scientists

Radiation Brain Moms
and Citizen Scientists

The Gender Politics of Food Contamination

after Fukushima AYA HIRATA KIMURA

DUKE UNIVERSITY PRESS *Durham and London* 2016

© 2016 Duke University Press
All rights reserved
Printed in the United States of America
on acid-free paper ∞
Designed by Amy Ruth Buchanan
Typeset in Minion by Westchester Publishing Services

Library of Congress Cataloging-in-Publication Data
Names: Kimura, Aya Hirata, [date] author.
Title: Radiation brain moms and citizen scientists : the
gender politics of food contamination after Fukushima /
Aya Hirata Kimura.
Description: Durham : Duke University Press, 2016. |
Includes bibliographical references and index.
Identifiers: LCCN 2016008607 (print)
LCCN 2016011248 (ebook)
ISBN 9780822361824 (hardcover : alk. paper)
ISBN 9780822361992 (pbk. : alk. paper)
ISBN 9780822373964 (e-book)
Subjects: LCSH: Fukushima Nuclear Disaster, Japan,
2011. | Food contamination—Japan. | Mothers—Japan. |
Japan—Social conditions—21st century.
Classification: LCC HV623 2011.F85 K56 2016 (print) | LCC
HV623 2011.F85 (ebook) | DDC 363.19/20820952—dc23
LC record available at http://lccn.loc.gov/2016008607

Cover art: A mother with her son living in Fukushima
City approximately 60 km away from the Fukushima
Daiichi nuclear plant. © 2012 Katsuo Takahashi for
Human Rights Watch. All rights reserved.

TO MY PARENTS

CONTENTS

ABBREVIATIONS

ABCC	Atomic Bomb Casualty Commission
ALARA	as low as reasonably achievable
Bq	becquerel
CRMO	citizen radiation-measuring organization
ECRR	European Commission of Radiological Risk
EU	European Union
IAEA	International Atomic Energy Agency
ICRP	International Commission on Radiological Protection
LDP	Liberal Democratic Party
MDC	minimum detectable concentration
MDS	Movement for Democratic Socialism
mSv	millisievert
NAZEN	Let's Abolish All Nuclear Reactors Right Now
NGO	nongovernmental organization
PRPC	practical radiation protection culture
PRV	provisionary regulatory value
RERF	Radiation Effects Research Foundation
RRC	radiation risk communicator
STS	science and technology studies
TEPCO	Tokyo Electric Power Corporation
WHO	World Health Organization
WiN	Women in Nuclear

PREFACE

It was the evening of March 12 Hawai'i time that a neighbor knocked on the door to let us know that a strong earthquake hit Japan. After making sure that my family and close friends were safe through the intermittent connection of phone and Skype, I watched in horror as the natural disaster turned into a nuclear disaster. The distance between Hawai'i (where I now live and teach) and Japan did little to ease the feelings of profound shock but also of responsibility to respond to this crisis. I wanted to "do something" like many of the interviewees in the book explained how they felt after the disaster, and for an academic, a research study to understand the human impacts seemed like the natural thing to do.

Nonetheless, I started this research with a lot of hesitation. Disaster capitalism seems to include disaster research, and the triple disaster—as the earthquake, tsunami, and nuclear accident in March 2011 came to be called—looked to be creating a gold rush of sorts for researchers and academic institutions. I did not want to be an opportunist who used someone else's tragedy as data for my research. I would also be conducting this research as an "expatriate researcher" (Soh 2008, 241–49), a "native" woman returning to her community to study it. While the interest of foreign scholars might be welcome as a sign of their (and the West's) unwavering friendship with Japan as the country faced enormous challenges partly rooted in the long-standing culture of Japanese "occidental longing" (Kelsky 2001, 7), being an expatriate researcher could be a liability. Being native to the society might be helpful, given my language fluency, adeptness at reading cultural cues, and existing social networks. But the expatriate researcher can be seen as not having a stake in the field site despite her lineage, as she has the privilege of leaving the place and the people whenever she wishes. In a time of nuclear crisis when the question of evacuation or continued settlement loomed large (and some wealthy people simply fled Japan for fear of contamination), I often felt a critical gaze on me from some Japanese for having the option to leave despite my nationality. However, the seemingly straightforward binary of insider-outsider fails to capture overlapping subjectivities and social relations of researchers. I tried to take my own ambiguous position as a productive space that joined both the helpful familiarity with the place and the people as well as a reflexive strangeness that motivated new and different kinds of questions.

I conducted this research not as a detached outsider, but as someone with a strong investment in justice and equality in Japan and elsewhere. My family ties and identity notwithstanding, the more important anchor for me is solidarity based on struggles against injustice. I want to see the reconstruction and rebuilding become more just and equitable for marginalized communities; I also think about the future accidents that might happen elsewhere, including in the United States, and how we might work to prevent them.

During the fieldwork, I often felt strong pressure to take a side: Either "food is risky" or "food contamination turned out not to be so serious." This book, however, tells neither a story of victimization nor a story of heroism, which might disappoint many readers, both within and outside of Japan. Nonetheless, I hope it offers critical insights into the layers of tensions and opportunities that exist in citizens' struggles in contamination cases.

ACKNOWLEDGMENTS

Writing this book was possible only with the willingness of the people
I interviewed for it. They are too many to list individually, but include all
those in the groups that advocated for safe school lunches and the leaders and volunteers at citizen radiation measuring organizations who shared
their stories with me with patience and open hearts. I enjoyed working
with Katano Yohei at Tottori University, who provided invaluable expertise on food systems and environmental politics in Japan. Doshisha
University's Global and Regional Studies Department became my insti-
tutional home during my fieldwork, and Matsuhisa Reiko and Futamura
Taro at Doshisha University and Yasutake Rumi at Konan Women's University were wonderful hosts. Hosokawa Komei at Kyoto Seika University helped me get in touch with some key informants. Hiraga Midori and
Momoe Oga were extremely helpful in conducting interviews in Japan.
I also thank the editor of *School Lunch Magazine*, Mochizuki Shoko, for
sharing her insight in regard to school lunch programs in Japan. Everett
Wingert in the Department of Geography at the University of Hawai'i
graciously helped create the maps in this book. Special thanks are due
also to Christine Yano, Jane Moulin, Allison Sterling Henward, Nicolas
Sternsdorff-Cisterna, and a reviewer for giving me great feedback. I am
especially thankful to Keiko Tanaka for numerous valuable suggestions.
Courtney Berger of Duke University Press gave astute comments on
many renditions of the project. Laurie Durand proofread many drafts
and did meticulous editing. For a research grant, I thank the National
Science Foundation's Science, Technology, and Society program. Any
opinions, findings, and conclusions or recommendations expressed in

this book are mine and do not necessarily reflect the views of the National Science Foundation.

In the space given to acknowledgments the writer is forgiven, I hope, for being a bit personal and self-indulgent, and I want to use it for expressing gratitude to my family. My parents—Ryoko and Masahiro Hirata—have been the best parents I could hope for, always supportive of whatever I have set out to do since childhood. I dedicate this book to them with my deepest gratitude for providing love and confidence. My sister, Miwa, whose son was still small when the accident happened, was an ardent observer and listener in the research process. I also want to thank my extended family members, particularly the Nakano clan in Kyoto, who took me and my family under their wing when we moved there for one year for the research. My parents-in-law, Keiko and Rihito Kimura, have supported my family in numerous ways, and they also connected me to important interviewees. Finally, my biggest thanks go to my partner, Ehito Kimura. With his generous heart, he has been an intellectual comrade and soul mate, encouraging me to take this journey, acting as a sounding board for ideas, and always willing to help.

My children, Isato and Emma, came to Japan with me for a year and endured my absence when I went off to different places for research. They remember that year as "when mama was on trips a lot." But even when I was away from them, they were never far from my thoughts. They were in my mind when I interviewed mothers and fathers who wondered if what was in the pot for dinner was contaminated and about feeling guilty for not being able to take their children to a cleaner place. I could not help thinking about my own children when I listened to interviewees talking about their families, which made me feel these other parents' pain and agony viscerally. It is for Isato and Emma—and for all children—that I wrote this book, in the hope that it will help make their future more sustainable and just.

Except for people in public offices, individuals' names are pseudonyms. For Japanese names, I followed the Japanese convention of putting the surname first, before the given name. The quotes from interviews in Japanese and from Japanese-language publications were translated by the author unless otherwise indicated.

INTRODUCTION

On March 12, 2011, Nomura Atsuko and her husband were glued to the
TV, watching the news from the blast at the Fukushima Daiichi Nuclear
Power Plant, which had been damaged by the massive earthquake and
tsunami that had just taken place. They were 150 miles away from Fukushima, well beyond the area that the government said had to be evacuated.
But as they watched the news coverage, Nomura-san (*san* is a Japanese
honorific) did not feel particularly safe.

Over the next few months, Nomura-san became increasingly concerned about the effects of radiation. Her lingering fear was confirmed
several months later, when her son's urine was tested and found to con-
tain radioactive cesium, albeit a small amount. She blamed herself for
believing, for even a second, the government's claims that food in general was not contaminated. The government had been insisting on a state
of normalcy and safety, chastising those with radiation concerns as irrational and antiscientific overreactions that were harmful to the national
economy. But she resolved to make sure no more radiation would get
into her son's body. Wanting to know the actual contamination levels
of the food she was cooking, and driven by the desire to protect other
children as well as her own, she and her friends established an organization to open a citizen-run station where people could bring their food to
have its level of contamination measured.[1] Such groups, which I call citizen radiation-measuring organizations (CRMOs), emerged across Japan
after the accident.

The Fukushima accident was arguably one of the most serious food
controversies in Japanese history. The government first admitted a food

safety threat on March 19, a week after the blast at the plant, following the discovery of contaminated vegetables and milk. But the extent of contamination was uncertain, and citizens highly doubted the government's willingness to make it transparent. It was in this context that citizen science, in various forms such as CRMOs, emerged as a central feature of postaccident food politics.[2]

Many saw the spread of CRMOs and other instances of citizen science as a sign of a rejuvenated activism in Japan that might destabilize the power of political and economic elites. Dubbed the nuclear village (*genshiryokumura*), the alliance of the utility industry, other business sectors, and technocrats constitutes the core of the Japanese polity. The utility industry's tendrils reach into various facets of the economy and society in Japan (Kainuma 2011). For instance, the manufacturing of reactors and their maintenance is an important business for the heavy equipment industry. Insurance and banking industries are the major stockholders of the utility companies. The utility industry also has a significant PR budget, which ties them to the media industry (Honma 2013). The strong push for nuclear power in Japan has also been entangled with the geopolitical interests of Japan and the United States: Japan must keep its nuclear weapons capacity to maintain a global strategic nuclear balance (Schreurs 2013).

The nuclear accident seemed to open a space to challenge the power of the nuclear village. Many citizen groups formed to measure radiation levels for themselves, contrary to pronouncements of safety. There were also several noteworthy demonstrations that brought tens of thousands of people into the streets. But today, the nuclear village remains largely intact, and it has not been held fully accountable for the accident. For instance, the government installed the new Basic Energy Plan in 2014, which was premised on restarting existing nuclear plants and even left open the possibility of building new ones despite citizens' desire to quickly phase out nuclear energy. As described in a *New York Times* article in 2014: "The country's organized opposition to nuclear power—which erupted in the months after the Fukushima accident into mass street rallies—has failed to materialize" (Tabuchi 2014).

What happened to those citizen scientists who challenged the picture of normalcy? Some scholars observed that citizen scientists actually failed to play a significant role in a larger antinuclear movement, or diverted the momentum away from radical politics. Political scientist

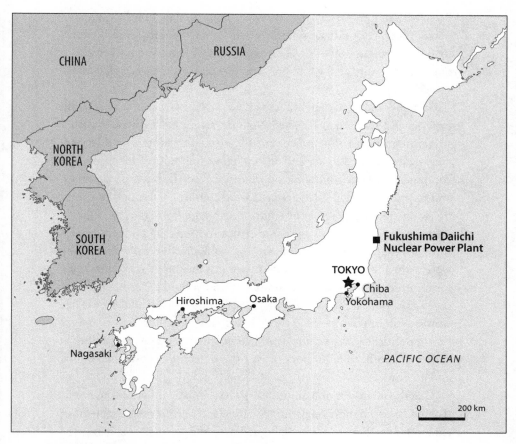

Map I.1 The location of the Fukushima Daiichi nuclear power plant.

Richard Samuels wrote, for instance, that "social mobilization was personified . . . in 'citizen scientists' who collected data on radioactivity in their neighborhoods. . . . Japanese citizens seemed *more concerned than outraged* during the first year after the disaster" (2013a, 132, emphasis added).

Samuels's image of depoliticized citizen scientists captures the jarring experience I had when I visited Nomura-san's CRMO. I had expected something like an NGO office, but the space felt more like a laboratory, neat and functional, and with a bare minimum of furniture and equipment (a table and chairs, a detector, a refrigerator, a computer, and plastic containers). No activists were coming in and out, nor were there any political flyers or brochures. Although housed in an unlikely place, in the corner of a large game center and separated only by panels from rows of game machines buzzing with mechanical music (they were using the space to save money on rent), the CRMO was remarkable for its atmosphere of extreme simplicity and solitude. Despite her outrage against the authorities for their "lies" and "propaganda," to use her words, Nomura-san seemed more like a diligent laboratory manager than a political activist—she would come into the office (they tellingly called it "mother's laboratory"), run the detector, record the results, and go home.

Like the members of Nomura-san's CRMO, many other citizen scientists also focused more on getting accurate and reliable measurements of contaminants than, say, organizing rallies, protests, or sit-ins. While the literature on citizen science and popular epidemiology has documented many cases of social movement activists skillfully utilizing scientific tools for social change, citizen science after the Fukushima accident seemed to exert taming effects on activism, as the "more concerned than outraged" citizenry apparently took to science instead of politics.

Because food was one of the few tangible ways in which the radiation threats became visible, and its circulation was not limited to the reactor's immediate vicinity, food could potentially have made an effective rallying point for social movements. Food is also an intimate commodity, which could have been a rich emotional resource for social movements to use to build affective connections among diverse groups of people. But radicalization through food politics did not take place in post-Fukushima Japan.

The understanding of post-Fukushima dynamics would be severely limited if it is simply seen as a case of effective government information control that silenced citizen scientists. My argument in this book is that the constraints for citizen scientists came from much broader forces of neoliberalism, scientism, and postfeminism. These forces reinforced notions of citizenship that largely excluded political activism, rendering activism inappropriate for an ideal citizen.

This book analyzes the complicated relationship between citizen science and politics in post-Fukushima Japan through the concept of food policing, which refers to the censoring of people's concerns about food safety in the name of science, risk analysis, and economy. An obvious example of food policing was the authorities' insistence that there was no health threat from food after the accident and criticism of people like Nomura-san. But the concept of food policing tries to capture the more insidious nature of social dynamics beyond government propaganda and to clarify their linkages to broader shifts in social policy, political economy, and gender relations. Food policing censors safety concerns not merely by public relations campaigns but more fundamentally by reinforcing the notion of the appropriate citizen-subject that is aligned with neoliberalism, postfeminism, and scientism. Good citizens are expected to act in accordance with dominant scientific knowledge and as rational economic beings, and to eat foods despite safety concerns so as not to disturb economic prosperity.

As Michelle Murphy (2012, 2) noted in her seminal book on the relationship between the US feminist movement and scientific practices, the complicated "entanglement" implicates women in the often problematic tendencies of the modern scientific paradigm. Because of the dual stereotypes of women as domestic and irrational, food policing particularly targets women as people who have a strong attachment to food issues and who tend to act out of deficient scientific knowledge. Food policing creates an environment where science emerges as a way to perform an ideal citizen-subject, particularly for women who have to compensate for their perceived weakness in technoscientific matters, while it constrains women from radicalizing, given the cultural dictum that science be value free and apolitical. The good neoliberal citizen-subject is someone who is personally responsible and constructive, and female citizens need to navigate carefully to be resourceful and scientifically enlightened. Female citizens are also supposed to act appropriately feminine, although such constraints tend to be invisible under the ideology of postfeminism, which presumes that women have already been emancipated and gender stereotypes vanquished.

These central findings of the book have significant implications for social struggles around environmental and food contamination beyond the case of the Fukushima accident. If citizen science becomes a means to perform a neoliberal, technical citizen, its radical political potential is likely to be lost. Contamination cases often involve the call for citizen participation and input, but what if the notion of "citizen" itself has significantly shifted? Redress of injustice from contamination is difficult when citizen mobilizations are constrained by prevailing preferences for neoliberal, postfeminist, and technical-rational identities.

My approach to post-Fukushima food contamination is rooted in science and technology studies' (STS') analyses of contemporary environmental pollution and contamination issues. Many scholars in this tradition have underscored the socially embedded ways in which contaminants become visible or invisible and in which they become socially controversial or rendered nonissues. In regard to the question that I posed above about the domestication and lack of social mobilization of citizen scientists, it is possible to argue that it was because contamination turned out to be negligible. This is a highly controversial issue, and this book does not intend to offer a definitive assessment of the extent of food contamination after the nuclear accident or its health impacts.[3] Instead of judging what the true state of contamination was and what the appropriate response should have been, I am more interested in the power relations that shaped dominant understandings of these issues: Who had the power to decide the right way to be concerned, and what shaped the way social institutions and citizens responded to the contamination? These are significant questions, as many contamination cases, including but not limited to radiation contamination, are inherently complex and riddled with scientific uncertainties. If society responds by food policing, it is difficult to have meaningful societal debates on how to respond to contamination and its systemic sources.

This book does not tell a triumphant story of citizen science facing down the authorities' propaganda to reveal contamination and danger. The story it tells is a fragmented one of food policing that tried to force silence and was cultivated not only by the elites but also by the people.

This is a story as well of how people, particularly women, turned to science to break the silence but were simultaneously constrained in politicizing science. Trying to understand such a messy picture will, I believe, shed light on the constraints on anticontamination activism and citizen science in contemporary societies.

Food Policing

Takeshita-san is a stylish woman in her forties who came to her interview with me on a bike wearing a pair of enamel high heels. She used to be a career-oriented woman, a *bari-kyari* (*bari* comes from *baribari*, which means "aggressively," and *kyari* for "career"), working in corporate public relations in Tokyo. When the earthquake hit, she was in her office working, where she stayed despite the strong jolts and many aftershocks. She had a son in preschool but figured that he would be safe there, so she worked late that day, and she tried to come to work on the following days.

Soon after the accident, the government started a national advertising campaign to calm growing fears about food contamination and to lessen the impact of what they called *fūhyōhigai* (harmful rumors), as consumer avoidance was reducing sales of food products from the affected area. In this Eat to Support campaign, the government disseminated the message that consumer avoidance caused enormous economic and social damage, and that food sold in the markets was safe. For instance, the government created a TV advertisement featuring TOKIO, a longtime popular singing group of five men. It started with a shot of one of the members eating a big rice ball, followed by the others biting into a whole cucumber, then an apple, a skewer of beef, and a tomato, all smiling happily. The voice-over said, "Today, all of Japan is closely connected through our good food and our pleasure in eating together. *Itadakimasu!* [Bon appétit]." This was followed by the slogan, "Let's continue to eat to support!" spoken in cheerful unison by the stars. The advertisement ended with an image of the logo for Food Action Nippon, which is a smiling figure with a red dot in the middle, invoking the national flag (see figure I.1). The choice of TOKIO, a group with a large female following, makes it clear that the message was targeted at female Japanese citizens.

In line with the government's campaign, one of Takeshita-san's first jobs after the accident was to counter fūhyōhigai in a marketing campaign

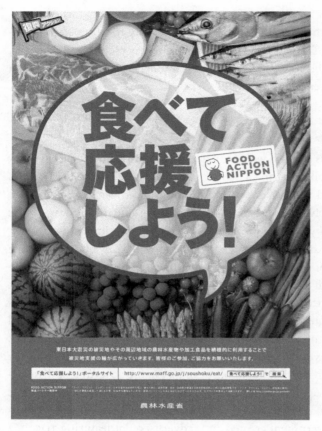

Figure I.1 A poster by Food Action Nippon. The text says, "Let's eat to support!" Source: Food Action Nippon, Ministry of Agriculture, Forestry and Fisheries.

for food from the affected area. Her company was going to start a project to bring children to a farm in Chiba Prefecture, which had suffered from declining sales due to its proximity to Fukushima. Takeshita-san had read online that some places in Chiba had been found to be hot spots of cesium contamination. When she was assigned the project, she brought the issue up with her boss. But he scolded her for worrying about it and did nothing to check on the safety of food from the farm. Another project assigned to her was to advertise a restaurant that featured Fukushima food as part of the Eat to Support campaign. Since the restaurant's clientele was families with children, she could not help but worry about the possibility of contaminated food. She gathered her courage again to mention the issue to her boss. His reaction was as cold as the previous time, and he told her that she should not be worried about such things when the government said that the food was generally safe. Feeling desperate, she even tried to talk to the higher management of her company. But the director treated her like she was out of her mind; she even cried in the office. And her colleagues did not sympathize with her at all either. She had been working full time for close to twenty years in the industry and had pioneered many projects as a woman. But now she felt isolated and ostracized. She quit her job and decided to join a group of mothers who later established a CRMO in her neighborhood.

One might argue that Takeshita-san was overreacting and that food contamination was well controlled and kept to a minimum. Indeed, the actual additional radiation exposure that each person might receive from food seemed to be contained below the government standards.[4] Setting aside for the moment the debate about whether the government standards were valid or not, and whether the sampling, frequency, and testing method were rigorous enough, the levels of contamination found continued to decrease. The government data showed that only 2.2 percent of rice, 3 percent of vegetables, and 20 percent of seafood tested in 2011 exceeded the government standards. The odds of contamination declined as time passed. In 2013, no tested rice or vegetables exceeded the standards, and only 4 percent of seafood tested did.[5]

This book does not evaluate whether Takeshita-san's response was logical or irrational. Rather, it points out that the way she was ostracized for raising the issue of contamination was reflective of a larger dynamic of food policing that worked to suppress societal debates over the issue. The questions mentioned above, about the uncertainties of the tests, standards, and underlying scientific knowledge, were actually fundamental rather than peripheral to the problem of radiation contamination. Food policing marginalized the need for collective and societal processes to make sense of radiation threats in an atmosphere of such profound uncertainty and complexity.

The concept of food policing takes a cue from the French philosopher Jacques Rancière and the contrast he draws between policing and politics.[6] In his reading, today's democratic societies rarely have real politics despite their nominal embrace of democracy; rather, policing is what proliferates, naturalizing and reinforcing the given boundaries for insti-tutions and citizens.[7] The way Takeshita-san was chastised for worrying about food contamination illuminates the force of such policing, which creates a society in which what one can sense, discuss, and problematize is already defined by the existing social order. Food policing involves the normalization of a certain level of risk with food as inevitable, impos-ing a particular view of reality and a prescription for the right kind of conduct. People's worries, concerns, and actions to lower food risk are censored in the name of science, risk analysis, and the economy.

This book examines the Japanese experience to highlight three char-acteristics of food policing and show why they have power in con-temporary society. The first characteristic is food policing's relationship with neoliberalism. Neoliberalism's advocacy of limited government, a free market, and individualism is paradoxically combined with a preoc-cupation with security and social order (Wacquant 2010). The concern with social order and economic recovery is particularly heightened in times of disaster and catastrophe (Tierney and Bevc 2010). Furthermore, in its quest for harmony and discipline in society, neoliberal policing makes civil society its partner. As Mitchell Dean says of the "liberal po-lice," it "employs techniques and agencies located within civil society rather than merely issuing regulations and thus must rely on a knowl-edge of economic, social and other processes outside the formal sphere of the state" (2002, 42). The way Takeshita-san was scolded by her colleagues, who she thought were her friends, is a good example of the insidious na-ture of policing, which works not always from above but sometimes from within civil society. Similarly, it is instructive to note that reactions by av-erage Japanese people to the authorities' Eat to Support campaign and fūhyōhigai criticism were more often than not enthusiastic rather than shocked or outraged. Instead of starting a movement to boycott certain products or to mobilize the electorate, many people seemed to be happy to "eat to support," believing the government pronouncement that what was sold in the markets needed to be deemed safe. How Japanese re-sponded to the nuclear accident was not always to engage in politics, but often to take part in policing.

Second, scientism is evident in food policing, with its central tenet that food decisions ought to be based on science and rational risk calcu-lation. Scientism refers to the reliance of regulatory policies on science at the exclusion of consideration over social-cultural factors and distributional effects (Moore et al. 2011). While scientism's influence varies in different countries (Jasanoff 2005), there has been a general increase in its strength (Moore et al. 2011). The advanced capitalist states are increasingly using science in their regulatory systems, normalizing it as the ultimate arbiter of policy issues (Jasanoff 2005).[8] Such scientization of governance has often resulted in the sidelining of democratic processes and the marginalization of ordinary citizens (Welsh and Wynne 2013). Food policing reflects this dynamic of scientism, which authorizes science to have the final word on food controversies, obfuscating their social and cultural roots and consequences.

Third, food policing is gendered. The demarcation of contamination as an exclusively scientific issue tends to exclude women, who are usually dismissed as weak on scientific issues. As Todd May has said, "there is no police order without the participation of the people, those people who are politically invisible, each in her proper space" (2008, 48); politics and science are not a "proper space" for women, particularly in Japan, where gendered segregation is still pervasive. For instance, in an international comparison of the ratio of women in national parliaments, Japan was 134th (8.1 percent), the lowest among the developed nations, while, for instance, Sweden's ratio is more than 40 percent and that of the United States, 18 percent (Inter-Parliamentary Union 2014). The gender gap is also salient in science in Japan. For instance, only about 25 percent of science and 10 percent of engineering undergraduate degrees are earned by women in Japan (Ministry of Economics, Trade, and Industry 2009).

Furthermore, under the effects of postfeminism and neoliberalism, in what Angela McRobbie (2009) calls the postfeminist gender settlement, women are increasingly considered to be economically mobile players in society but are still required to conform to hegemonic femininity and behave in ways that are nonthreatening to men. This new sexual contract also lets women have power as long as they do not question the main assumption of postfeminism—that structural inequality is no longer a problem. In this gender dynamic, women are allowed to become politically vocal only to a limited degree, while radical activism is policed as incongruent for these aspirational and feminine citizen-subjects.

Of course, the three social forces—scientism, neoliberalism, and postfeminism—are not separate, but mutually constitutive. Neoliberalism's impact on science has been profound; it has reduced public funding for research and increased the need for private resources and the commodification of research through intellectual property protection. Neoliberalism also entails privatization and commodification of biophysical resources, which privileges technocratic methods of their valuation and management. Furthermore, not only is science neoliberalized, but neoliberalism is scientized (Pellizzoni and Ylönen 2012); now ubiquitous, corporate self-governance (instead of government regulation) tends to rely on technical parameters and ignore distributive and cultural issues. Freer trade under neoliberalism is facilitated by the harmonization of standards and regulations, resulting in the proliferation and expansion of the power of transnational technical bodies that set global benchmarks and standards based on technical and scientific frameworks (Moore et al. 2011), as in the case of radiation protection standards.

The entanglements of neoliberalism and scientization are beginning to be theorized in STS, but this book points out another element in this coproduction: postfeminism. Neoliberalism promotes a masculinized, rational, calculating, and risk-taking subjecthood, which in turn facilitates neoliberalization (Ferber and Nelson 2009; Griffin 2007). Neoliberalism benefits from the postfeminist discourse that features have-it-all women as a marker of the enlightenment and meritocracy of the market-based system (McRobbie 2009; Rottenberg 2014). While better-off women are groomed to be entrepreneurial and productive agents in the global economy, less privileged women tend to take the brunt of the impacts of neoliberal cuts in social services.

Scientism and postfeminism are also mutually constitutive. Western science has historically developed in a way that privileges male perspectives and experiences, and the increasing power of science has tended to exacerbate male power in academia, medicine, and bureaucracy. Yet scientism often works to fortify the notion that policy debates are gender neutral and simply technical, while portraying the historic exclusion of women as no longer relevant. Scientism also implies a value-free meritocracy in line with the postfeminist idea that we already live in a meritocratic world free of stereotypes and discrimination.

Nowhere but in the idea of the citizen, implicit in food policing, are the combined influences of these dynamics more salient. A proper citizen-subject is increasingly understood to be a rational, aspirational, and appropriately gendered one who would understand contamination primarily as scientific risk issue to be handled without disturbing existing social, economic, and gender orders.

To be sure, food is only one of the many contamination issues that became highly policed in post-Fukushima Japan. For instance, information disclosure on airborne radiation was insufficient, leading many local groups to collect and share test data (Morita, Blok, and Kimura 2013); contaminated debris—which accumulated partly from the decontamination work—had to be disposed of or stored somewhere, triggering similar safety questions and severe sanctions against the opposition (see, for instance, "Garekishorihantainiwa 'Damare'" 2011); and the lifting of evacuation orders by the government, which urged residents to return to their homes in contaminated areas, also drew criticisms and counter-criticisms ("Fukushimagenpatsujiko" 2015; Shirabe 2013). This book focuses on food policing, however, as food is increasingly a focal point for social mobilization around the world (Alkon and Agyeman 2011; Allen 2007; Gottlieb and Joshi 2010; Windfuhr and Jonsén 2005). Food is a powerful lens through which to examine broader social injustices, economic stratification, and environmental sustainability, and the concept of food policing enables focused analyses of the constraints on citizens' ability to engage in these issues.

The empirical material in the book is limited to case studies in Japan after the Fukushima accident, but my hope is that the book's theoretical and conceptual insights can be extended beyond them to understand broader dynamics surrounding contamination, citizen science, and food politics. Reinforced by and in turn reinforcing neoliberalism's prioritization of economic growth and its emphasis on personal responsibility and prevailing scientism, food policing is a chronic feature of food safety controversies in advanced capitalist societies. Social controversies around genetically modified organisms and bovine spongiform encephalopathy (mad cow disease) have involved similar patterns of safety concerns being condemned and ridiculed as antiscience, harmful to the economy, and costing jobs.

Many cases of food contamination are riddled with profound uncertainty. But if food policing is allowed to dominate the societal response to it, little space remains for contradictory scientific views, opinions, and values to be expressed to form a basis for figuring out social and political, not necessarily scientific, solutions to the situation. It is because food policing results in the annihilation of dissensus that it is not ultimately helpful in rehabilitating food systems after contamination scandals.

Citizen Science and Its Politics

Would citizen science be a way to counter food policing? Olga Kuchinskaya (2014), in her book on the Chernobyl accident, discussed how the government and international and domestic scientists were implicated in the production of the invisibility of radiation, and wondered how a robust civil society in the case of Fukushima might make it easier to make radiation visible. From this perspective, the difference between Chernobyl and Fukushima was that the former happened in an authoritarian state and the latter in a free and democratic society. In such a milieu, citizen science can be expected to create a subversive infrastructure for making radiation visible, laying the foundation for social action. In fact, after the Fukushima accident, there were many grassroots activities that could be understood as citizen science. Many people started measuring contaminants in the air and sharing the results online (Morita, Blok, and Kimura 2013), as well as establishing CRMOs to help citizens screen their own food.

However, the political potential of citizen science is contingent upon complex social and historical dynamics, and varying sets of constraints as well as enablers exist even in the case of a liberal democratic society. Whether citizen science results in radical criticism of the powerful institutions and hegemonic discourses requires in-depth empirical analyses. Among Japanese studies scholars, different evaluations of post-Fukushima citizen scientists have emerged. On the one hand, observers like sociologist Daniel Aldrich, who studies Japanese politics, took citizen scientists as an example of a "renaissance in civil society" (2013, 264). On the other hand, as mentioned earlier, Richard Samuels suggested that citizen scientists like those in the CRMOs exemplify a domesticated civil society that failed to achieve substantial political changes. Japanese citizens expended a great deal of energy in testing food and air for cesium concentrations, but that kind of citizen science activity diverted them from real politics.

In the STS debate on citizen science, too, its political potential is increasingly under scrutiny. From impacts of pesticides (Kleinman and

Suryanarayanan 2012) to genetically modified foods (Kinchy 2012), citizen groups and laypeople are doing their own research to fill gaps in knowledge on food safety and quality, and there are many reasons why they are valuable as important contributors to society. Citizen scientists might possess local knowledge that experts might not have access to (Corburn 2005). Science activity by lay people is also seen as a way to enhance the science literacy of the public, improving their understanding of science. Citizen science might also expose values and hidden assumptions naturalized in official science (Epstein 1998). By doing so, it can also open new lines of inquiry and set new agendas that might not emerge if science is left to experts (Hess 2007). Some also see an inherent virtue in citizen science in that it embodies participatory and democratic orientations, critical in a democratic society (Fischer 2000; Irwin 1995).

However, while we can celebrate citizen science as an instance of the democratization of science, it is nonetheless important to analyze it in relation to a larger political context of neoliberalization. In the United States, for instance, scholars have noticed that the increase in citizen environmental monitoring has occurred in tandem with neoliberalization. Because of government budget cuts, particularly in what is often seen as unproductive areas such as environmental protection, environmental monitoring is increasingly relegated to nonprofit community groups. Therefore, what political geographer Rebecca Lave (2012) calls "extramural" science is now a common feature of governance in the age of neoliberalism.

Neoliberalism's impact is also evident in who counts as a citizen in citizen science. Neoliberalism comes with a particular normative understanding of the citizen-subject (Ong 2006). Its celebration of market principles and economic efficiency naturalizes the assumption of *homo economicus*, a rational and rent-seeking human being. It is also linked to what Burchell (1996), following Foucault's work on governmentality, called responsibilization, in which one is interested in and held responsible for the care of oneself. This discourse produces a particular kind of subjectivity that emphasizes self-regulation and self-care. Therefore, citizen science can be seen as a part of responsibilization—putting pressure on citizens to take responsibility for their own well-being and hence driving them to collect data that are necessary for their health and safety.

Neoliberal citizens are also expected to contribute to societal well-being by their engagement with civil society. It is intriguing to notice that there is intrinsic tension between neoliberalism and the concept of the citizen that is articulated by classical political theories. The neoliberal model of homo economicus presupposes the individualism of self-interested humans acting autonomously on rational calculations, while in the classical ideal, citizens engage in dialogue, cooperation, and the collective pursuit of the good life. The tension is resolved in the concept of civil society, which, perhaps predictably, has become popular since the 1980s, when neoliberalism was starting to flex its muscles in the advanced capitalist countries. The civil society as a discourse suggested that if neoliberalism molded people to be self-interested, aggressive profit maximizers and resulted in the rending of the social fabric, the remedy was to be found in civil society, which could patch it back together and function as a "flanking, compensatory mechanism for the inadequacies of the market mechanism" (Jessop 2002, 455). Therefore, some scholars interpreted the proliferation of NGOs not as the strengthening of democracy but as a telltale sign of neoliberalism: the "relinquish[ing] by the state of the obligations to provide citizenship rights" (Yudis 1995, cited in Fischer 2008, 7). Neoliberal citizens are then to take part not only in the market, but also in civil society, providing services to fellow citizens that help to maintain social cohesion, harmony, and control.

It is also important to notice how the work of civil society is often coded as feminine. Women are considered to be engaged in nurturing and caring activities in addition to productive economic activities. This feminine marking is somewhat counterintuitive from the point of view of the historical development of citizenship, which was restricted to men in many societies. But neoliberalism codes economic activity as masculine, as Penny Griffin pointed out: "By presenting the 'definitively human' activity of economic production as a characteristically masculine activity, neo-liberal discourse consigns both non-men and non-masculine persons to the spheres of non-productive or reproductive labor, where they are thus situated outside the society of male producers" (2007, 233). Because neoliberal discourse designates the "productive" sphere a male sphere, nonproductive citizen activities are read as appropriate to the female. In the Japanese context too, women have been historically active in nonremunerative charity and social welfare projects such as parent-teacher associations (Mackie 2003).

This literature leaves important questions unanswered: To what extent does citizen science go beyond individualistic acts of self-care or projects of domesticated civil society? What kind of citizen is implied in citizen science in a specific historical context? How does the gendered nature of civil society influence the politicization of citizen science? Because of science's cultural separation from politics, citizen science might be an ideal civil society activity under neoliberalism: a way to perform being constructive and helpful citizen-subjects who resourcefully take care of themselves.[9]

Gendered Constraints on Contamination Activism

Women are often at the forefront of environmental and health-related struggles in communities. Food in particular is historically considered women's domain in many societies; women are usually more concerned about its quality and safety, and they tend to join related social movements. The aftermath of the Fukushima accident saw a similar pattern, where many more women were concerned about food contamination than men, and many women took the lead in doing citizen science, including CRMOS.

Constraints on women's activism against contamination are complex and multifaceted, but this book examines three of them in particular to elucidate the historically specific and gendered dynamics of policing. The first is the stereotype of women as weak on technoscientific matters and more emotional than rational. Such stereotypes and the scientized view of contamination problems tend to compel women to resort to science in demanding decontamination and the rehabilitation of contaminated systems. But at the same time, in order to count as legitimate science, its boundary with politics needs to be carefully maintained, exerting a strong taming effect on female citizen scientists.

The second is the postfeminist gender settlement, a "new sexual contract" theorized by Angela McRobbie (2009, 54), that nominally grants women equal status with men while keeping the assumption of postfeminism—that systemic oppression of women is gone and that activism is no longer necessary. The trade-off is that the settlement gives women an entry to the public sphere, but only on the condition of complacency with the existing power structure and of adherence to hegemonic femininity. Under this settlement, then, women can address contamination issues only insofar as they act as proper women (such as mothers and docile, feminine citizens). Furthermore, because the idea of postfeminism assumes the existence of a meritocracy without gender biases, women's empowerment becomes the responsibility of individual women. This incentivizes women to play the game deftly rather than question the rules of the game, seemingly aligning women's interests with those in power. Criticisms of the power structure of society at a systemic level become extremely difficult.

The third constraint on women's activism is the increase in care demands under neoliberalism. Care work—bearing children and taking care of them, and caring for the sick, the disabled, and the elderly—is heavily feminized (Glenn 2000). Neoliberalism's cuts in social spending privatize the social work of care to the market (where it is also heavily feminized) or to female members of families and communities. The well-to-do might be able to purchase care services on the market, but most women have to personally shoulder the increasing care demands. The gendered, racialized, and classed decomposition of labor rights under neoliberalism also means that women are often at the bottom of the workforce, forcing them to patch together different wage-earning or informal activities for survival. As Rebecca Dolhinow (2014) observed about Mexican women's activism, the double and triple demands of being a wife/mother, worker, and activist can easily be overwhelming, with the last often dropping out of the equation. Similarly, contamination issues are likely to be only one among many of the problems that face these women who have to juggle multiple responsibilities for personal, family, and community survival. Sacrificing other care needs for activism might not be practical for many women in such environments.

On the other hand, the same forces of neoliberalism, scientism, and postfeminism make it alluring for women to be complacent about contamination issues. Risk is the increasingly dominant approach to hazards and contamination cases in contemporary society, often propelled by scientism and further cemented by the neoliberal ethos of rational management. While women are said to be more risk averse and ill equipped to have a rational risk paradigm, a new set of global, economic, and social circumstances are making new demands on women to have a more positive relationship with risk. Under neoliberalism, the idea of risk is increasingly understood as a potential economic value; risk is something that economically astute actors can leverage for future return. Furthermore, as anthropologist Megan Moodie (2013) observed, this understanding of risk marks people who take risk (risk takers) as agentic subjects with courage and leadership. This understanding of risk as value/agency allures women to be active not as radical activists against risk, but rather as risk takers who deal with contamination as scientific and economized risk.

In summary, complex layers of constraints on women may hinder them from mobilizing against and challenging environmental contamination, particularly under the neoliberal and postfeminist ideologies that subject women to limiting and disabling notions of citizen-subjecthood. Women are also required to act in line with hegemonic femininity to count as legitimate and appropriate citizens. Additionally, neoliberal cuts in social spending and public programs increase the care demands on women who have to juggle many responsibilities to ensure the survival and wellness of their family and community members, reducing the time, energy, and resources available for radical activism. Furthermore, gendered policing increases the pressure for women to resort to science, but as a project detached from politics. Combined, then, scientism, postfeminism, and neoliberalism cajole women toward demobilization and depoliticization.

Contamination Politics in Japan

Japan has often been celebrated as a showcase of ecological moderniza-tion, with its avowed pursuit of stringent environmental regulations and an efficient and sustainable economy.[10] The most notorious pollution cases, such as Minamata mercury poisoning, itai-itai disease caused by cadmium, and Yokkaichi asthma, are usually seen as relics of the past, an unfortunate byproduct of the rapid industrialization that occurred after World War II.[11] Contemporary Japan has been considered an exem-plary green nation, with rigorous regulations and smart industries (Bar-rett 2005).[12] Nuclear energy fits uneasily into this discourse of ecological modernization. As in the United States, nuclear energy has increasingly been promoted in Japan as a climate-friendly energy source that is more sustainable than coal and oil.

Japanese have been long wary of nuclear power not only because of its association with the atomic bombs of World War II but also due to inter-national and domestic accidents.[13] Different types of antinuclear groups existed before the Fukushima accident, from the Socialist and Com-munist parties and labor unions to housewives in urban areas (Cavasin 2008). Many local communities have risen up to oppose nuclear power plants in their neighborhoods as well (Aldrich and Dusinberre 2011).

Overall, however, the antinuclear movement has had little success in opposing nuclear power.

Various reasons for this failure can be suggested. Japanese environmental organizations tend to have much smaller resource bases and to be less professionalized than Western environmental organizations. The movement has also suffered from internal fractures within organizations, particularly in the Socialist and Communist parties. Local opposition to nuclear power plants has tended to be suppressed by the political and economic muscle of the utility industry and the government, which injects large subsidies to appeal to economically deprived host communities. More broadly, nuclear power embodies environmental injustice, where the benefits of power accrue to the private sector and urban populations while the cost is disproportionately borne by impoverished host communities and marginalized workers who actually expose themselves to radiation even in nonaccident situations (Aldrich 2010; Hasegawa 1995; Kainuma 2011).

This book suggests the increasingly important role of science and women in both citizen mobilization and countermobilization by the authorities. The scientization of activism and its implications has not been analyzed in depth in the Japanese studies literature. In Japan's antinuclear movement, citizen science has played an important role, but its interpretation is usually different from the usual STS definition. The phrase "citizen scientist" (shiminkagakusha) in the Japanese context usually has meant scientists outside the elite establishment who work with laypeople. Some of these scientists have played an important role in the antinuclear movement, including those who established the Citizens' Nuclear Information Center and the People's Research Institute on Energy and Environment (Cavasin 2008, 67). This book focuses on the role of a different kind of Japanese citizen scientist, regular citizens without scientific qualifications who rose up to question the picture of normalcy and safety imposed by the authorities, and asks what it means that many resorted to science as a form of political challenge.

This book also analyzes women's role in contamination politics, particularly in relation to the changing gender order in contemporary Japan. Historically, many women have been active in antipollution cases and in the antinuclear movement. Food-related scandals have also brought many women into public debates, driven by the perceived affinity between women and food preparation and feeding (Kimura 2011). Existing literature has addressed some of the complex ways in which traditional gender stereotypes have both constrained and enabled women's activism. This book argues that the contemporary hypervisibility of women is a similarly double-edged sword, a problematic product of postfeminism and neoliberalism. Paraded as icons of economic mobility and social progressiveness, women are required to perform being a particular kind of citizen who is docile, feminine, and future oriented. This book examines women's roles, both as citizen scientists but also as risk communicators who work with the nuclear village to disseminate what is constructed as the scientifically correct view of radiation threats.

The Postfeminist Gender Settlement in Japan

Postfeminism is not a coherent ideology or a social movement but a term used to describe an increasingly widespread discourse that suggests the irrelevance of feminism under the assumption that gender equality is already achieved. Feminist scholars have understood postfeminism as part of a backlash against feminist mobilizations, given the tenacity of sexism despite formal codification of gender equality. The notion of postfeminism might seem even more incongruent with the situation in Japan, which in terms of gender equality seems to be farther behind the United States. For instance, the World Economic Forum's (2014) gender equality ranking put Japan at 104th out of 142 countries (while the United States was twentieth). Women's literacy rates and health outcomes are excellent in Japan, but other indicators—such as political and economic participation—tend to be among the worst in developed countries.

Japanese feminism has a long and varied history with diverse groups focusing on different issues, including legal codification of gender equality, educational reform, and solidarity with women in other Asian countries, particularly on the issue of sexual violence and militarized prostitution during World War II. Perhaps the most visible and institutionalized successes were in the 1980s and 1990s, including the ratification of the Convention on the Elimination of All Forms of Discrimination against Women and the establishment of the Equal Employment Opportunity Law in 1985, the establishment of the Office of Gender Equality in 1994, and the adoption of the Basic Law for a Gender-Equal Society in 1999 (Kobayashi 2004).

These policy advances triggered a backlash. One notable example was the controversy around the concept of *jendā furī* (gender free), which was used to denote gender equality in many policy programs, but was subsequently misrepresented by conservatives as an extremist concept that denied sex differences and facilitated radical sex education (Wakakuwa and Fujimura-Fanselow 2011; Yamaguchi 2014). There have also been efforts to reassert the centrality of the so-called traditional family, such as the establishment of the National Movement to Restore Family and Community Links in Support of Child Rearing in 2006 by Prime Minister Koizumi Junichiro and the Council for Japan Supporting Children and Families by Prime Minister Abe Shinzo (Wakakuwa and Fujimura-Fanselow 2011). Such backlash exists side by side with seemingly pro-women policies. The jarring picture was crystallized in Prime Minister Abe Shinzo's declaration in 2013 that he aimed to create a "society in which women shine," which he dubbed "womenomics" (Cabinet Office 2013c).

Coming from a politician who has long taken antifeminist positions (Wakakuwa and Fujimura-Fanselow 2011, 346), Abe's womenomics is a paradigmatic example of the postfeminist gender settlement. Calls for better work-life balance and expansion of maternity leave and child care support seem at first glance like women-friendly policies, and certainly many women would be glad to have them. Yet it is important to notice how womenomics reflects neoliberal economic pressure. Neoliberalization in Japan, as in other cases, is a complex process that is not without tensions and is quite malleable (Ong 2006). Particularly in the agricultural sector, the Japanese government has been critiqued for protectionist policies and the lack of willingness to introduce market-based reforms. The degree to which free market, free trade principles have changed policies is quite mixed. Nonetheless, after the late 1980s, the Japanese government felt the need to radically restructure the postbubble economy and undertook various neoliberal reforms including administrative reforms, welfare spending cuts, and privatization of railways and telecommunications. International pressure—particularly from the United States—also mounted to open up key markets such as financial and agricultural industries (Tiberghien 2014). The long-ruling Liberal Democratic Party (LDP)—which has been in power since 1955 with only sporadic interruptions—shifted toward favoring neoliberal policies despite resistance from its traditional constituents. The Koizumi administration (2001–2006) accelerated neoliberal reform to an unprecedented degree.

The Democratic Party, which took power between 2009 and 2011, was more critical of neoliberalism, but the LDP regained power in 2012 under Abe (Tiberghien 2014). Womenomics was part of his Abenomics, an aggressive economic platform for the revival of Japan. As Abe explained, the rationale behind womenomics was "the more the advance of women in society is promoted, the higher the growth rate becomes" (Cabinet Office 2013c).

Gestures toward women by conservative politicians like Abe have been driven in part by the realization that alienating women could be suicidal in elections (Kunihiro 2011, 370). But the neoliberal courting of women as a workforce—and a female workforce is still cheaper and more flexible as a reserve—also factored in the celebration of female power. Feminist scholars have pointed out that the Japanese government's push for a gender equality program has been motivated by the need to increase the labor force in the context of low fertility rates and the rapid aging of society (Yamaguchi 2014). It is pronatalist and neoliberal needs that motivated the conservative call for a greater role for women.

Neoliberalism seems to share the sensibility of liberal feminism in its emphasis on individuals as opposed to family as the smallest social unit. Given the confines of the traditional family, *ie*, which is often described as the entrapment of women, the individualist rhetoric of neoliberalism can sound feminist and might be seductive to many Japanese women (Alexy 2011). However, the concept of the postfeminist gender settlement reminds us that while the leash might be loosened it will not be released; women must be careful not to transgress too much, as hegemonic femininity and the heterosexual nuclear family remain linchpins of the conservative imagination of Japanese nationhood.

Structure of the Book

The book is divided into two broad sections. Chapters 1 and 2 examine the dynamics of the food policing that unfolded after the Fukushima nuclear reactor accident, while chapters 3, 4, and 5 examine potential challenges to food policing by regular citizens, particularly women.

Chapter 1 analyzes food policing through the discourse of fūhyōhigai and its gendered mechanisms. Originally designed to help food producers gain compensation for reduced sales due to the fear of contamination, the concept had a wider influence, often equating consumer worries with irrational fearmongering. As evident in the post-Fukushima neologism "radiation brain mom," the implicit target of the fūhyōhigai policing was women, understood as having an irrational "radiation brain," being anti-science, and overreacting. With its strong shaming effects, such food policing made many women's struggles with contamination a private problem that had to be dealt with in a highly secretive manner. Ironically, helping hands came from disaster capitalism, which offered products and services catering to the unmet needs of concerned consumers, but those who were not able to afford them were left out of this world of commodified safety. The neoliberal privatization of struggles with contamination under food policing raises the issue of class stratification.

Scientism in neoliberalism has made risk the primary frame for contamination issues, and chapter 2 examines gendered demands on citizens to take risks and communicate risks to fellow citizens. Specifically, the chapter examines risk communication as a facet of food policing by looking at how the Japanese government, the nuclear industry, and international nuclear organizations engaged in a public relations campaign in the name of scientific risk communication. The chapter suggests that an important modality of food policing is increasingly community based and feminized. Departing from the traditional expert-led model, risk communication today takes a participatory approach and frequently makes women the messengers as well as the targets. The "correct" kind of understanding of radiation was cultivated from the ground up and in a seemingly democratic manner, implicating women as important partners in this policing process.

Chapters 3, 4, and 5 examine how people responded to food policing, not through the market as in chapter 1, but by collective actions, particularly using science as a tool, and how they are shaped by postfeminism and neoliberalism. Chapter 3 examines the case of the safe school lunch movement (which was highly feminized), which demanded the government ensure the safety of the public school lunch program after the Fukushima accident. Food policing and the charge of fūhyōhigai made it difficult for women in the movement to speak up against the government position that no special measures were necessary in school lunch programs. This chapter describes three strategies that the women activists in the safe school lunch movement used, emphasizing science, motherhood, and hegemonic femininity. Women activists in the movement framed their demands around good science and testing, and also tried to authenticate their voices by emphasizing their identities as mothers and drawing on still-strong images of hegemonic femininity. Situating these three strategies in the context of neoliberalism, scientism, and the post-feminist gender settlement, I explore the extent to which the strategies were enabling as well as disabling of women's activism.

Chapters 4 and 5 discuss another instance of citizen science, the CRMOs. Chapter 4 gives a profile of CRMOs in Japan, describing their origin, structure, membership, and testing achievements. The chapter's emphasis is on CRMOs' political potential, however, and it asks whether CRMOs constituted activities of neoliberal citizens, or was part of an emergent food politics contra policing. The answer to the question of who can be a citizen in citizen science in contemporary Japan seems to be "not many people." In addition to neoliberal and postfeminist constraints on the idea of proper citizenship, post-Fukushima Japan saw a surge in radical left groups that made CRMOs highly wary of potential hijacking and the stigma of being associated with them. The space of the legitimate citizen became smaller and smaller, compelling many people to use science as a means to distance themselves from politics. But this does not mean that citizen science was completely depoliticized. With the concept of measuring on the margin, I argue that CRMOs sought to do politics by science, albeit in a highly constrained manner.

Chapter 5 continues to analyze CRMOs and asks questions regarding their precariousness. Three years after the accident, many of them were struggling to remain open and some had already closed down. Food policing must be understood as part of a larger landscape of neoliberalization and simultaneous erosion of citizenship entitlements and economic volatility. I identify the gendered care burden under neoliberalism as one of the reasons for the challenges facing many CRMOs. In addition, the chapter examines the temporality of contaminants constructed under neoliberalism and how forward-looking, aspirational neoliberal governmentality made a particular temporal understanding of radioactive materials salient.

Overall, the book critically examines the role of food policing in social responses to contamination and technoscientific disaster, as well as citizen mobilization in countering it. I situate the interplay between contamination and social responses at the intersection of scientism, neoliberalism, and postfeminism. The examination of food politics after the Fukushima accident helps us discern the dynamics where these forces are making new demands on women as scientifically rational, resourceful, and aspirational citizens. When contamination is turned into risk under scientism, and risk into the signs of agency and value under neoliberalism, the allure for citizens to condone it is formidable, particularly for women who are now endowed with nominal equality to realize their economic potential. Women are to take up technoscience as well as its underlying scientific rationality, and to engage with risk in a dual sense—to think of contamination through the rational risk paradigm as well as to take risks as savvy and aspirational economic actors.

On the surface, science and women seem to constitute potentially powerful forces against food policing. Ultimately, the book shows how they are significantly constrained by the limiting normative parameters for citizens, women, and politics.

ONE

"Moms with Radiation Brain"

Gendered Food Policing in the Name of Science

Kobayashi Akiko is a married working mother in her midthirties whose son was six years old when the Fukushima accident happened. She lived in Kanagawa Prefecture, south of Tokyo, which was 150 miles away from the troubled reactors and said to be safe according to the government. But the accident nonetheless made her very wary of radiation contamination, and she fled southward with her son immediately after she saw the news of the blast from the nuclear reactors. Because of work and school, among other reasons, it was not feasible for her to relocate permanently, so they came back home after a week. But nervous about her son's health, she decided to buy only food from the southern parts of Japan, avoiding anything from the northeast and eastern regions. She thought about joining a consumer cooperative famous for its strict food safety standards, but decided not to because she heard that they did not let their customers choose where their vegetables came from. Whenever she went grocery shopping, she looked at the details of each product's label to make sure it was not from the Tōhoku region. If a product's provenance was not clearly indicated on the label, she wouldn't buy it. While she had been an avid supporter of *chisan-chishō*, or local food movements, she started buying soy milk and other food products from Costco because they were from the United States, and she felt they were safer. She tried to avoid seafood from the affected areas too, but this was still a bit worrisome to her since she learned that the place of origin labeling for seafood products was quite ambiguous. She was not sure about her brown rice, either. Brown rice was said to be richer in nutrients but also more likely to have a higher contamination level than polished rice. "It has all become confusing," she said. "It is really stressful every day."

Kobayashi-san was one of the many mothers who have tried their best to avoid contaminated food in the aftermath of the Fukushima accident. The government and nuclear experts failed to provide information about food contamination in a timely and comprehensive manner. In the void that was created by the inability and unwillingness of experts to provide clear guidelines, laypeople began to cobble together bits of information and devise their own strategies in a desperate search for ways to mitigate radiation threats.

It is not a coincidence that it is mothers' stories that we have to narrate to understand the day-to-day struggles with food contamination threats. Domestic responsibilities are highly feminized, including daily preparation of food for one's family. After the nuclear accident, mothers devised various strategies to address potential harm from radioactive fallout from the troubled nuclear reactors—they avoided food from the affected areas, changed where they shopped for their food, and tried to cook in a way that would reduce the contamination. They also tried to get hold of detectors to measure the actual contamination levels of their food.

Rather than being commended as dutifully exercising their maternal responsibilities, these mothers were harshly condemned as irrational, emotional, and shameful. Despite the centrality of food in typical understandings of proper motherhood, the mothers who tried to cook uncontaminated food were not praised for their actions. Instead, the notion of *fūhyōhigai* (harmful rumors) was invoked to construe these concerned mothers as dangerous fearmongers. A compound of *fūhyō* (rumors) and *higai* (damages), the term refers to damage from the decline in sales of products that were regarded as contaminated with radiation. The connotation is that consumer avoidance of food is baseless: "subjectively considering food or products as unsafe without any scientific basis" (Sekiya 2011, 86), according to one expert on fūhyōhigai. Sometimes a more pointed term, "radiation brain mom," was used to deride these concerned mothers as hysterical and irrational. Avoiding foods from the affected areas, or even just expressing concerns about food safety, was understood less as maternal dedication to the health of one's family than as a lack of rationality, patriotism, and sympathy for the affected areas.

Drawing on feminist science and technology studies, I situate this sanctioning of mothers in a wider history of women's struggles related to scientific uncertainty and how their actions to respond to it often face social disapproval. Embedded in widespread gender stereotypes and deploying the full affective force of shame and guilt, fūhyōhigai constituted a critical power of the regime of food policing that was convenient for the elites who wanted to maintain the façade of normality after the accident. Seen as irrational or even discriminatory and prejudiced, mothers faced not only uncertainty about invisible contamination, but also social sanctions against their efforts to make sense of it.

Contaminated Food

The Fukushima nuclear accident caused a significant release of radioactive materials, and within a week of the earthquake, reports of contaminated food started to appear. On March 19, the government announced that it had found contaminated food, and subsequently ordered the governors of four prefectures to suspend shipments of spinach and milk. The contamination was not limited to Fukushima. In the same week, spinach from Takahagi City (Ibaraki Prefecture, 80–120 km away from the plants) had 15,020 Bq/kg of iodine 131, and similarly high values were found in spinach from other parts of Ibaraki Prefecture. Social anxiety increased as the media began to report contamination ("More and More Food Found above Standards" 2011; "Twenty-Five out of Forty-Five Fukushima Vegetables above Radioactive Standards" 2011).

Discoveries of contamination continued through the year: By January 2012, 1,048 cases of contamination had been detected by prefectural governments out of 89,786 samples (Ministry of Health, Labor, and Welfare 2012), and more than eighty government orders had been issued to stop shipments of food based on the Special Measures on Nuclear Disaster Act (Radiation Council 2012).[1]

But even this long list, many believed, was only partial, and there were several reasons for their suspicions. First, many people felt that the government was testing an insufficient number of samples. Only 16,829 tests were conducted in the first six months after the accident (Endo 2012, 84). In comparison, Belarus was reported to conduct 30,000 tests per day (Onuma 2013).

Furthermore, the government's criteria of what was contaminated and what was not depended upon what it started calling provisionary regulatory values (PRV). The Food Sanitation Act, which sets most of

Japan's food safety standards, did not have any standards for radiation. The government scrambled to come up with standards that would guide their disaster response, and adopted the values they found in a report by the Nuclear Safety Commission, which they called PRVs ("provisionary" because they were meant to be temporary until formal standards were set).[2] These PRVs were, for cesium, 300 Bq/kg for drinking water, milk, and other dairy products and 500 Bq/kg for other foods. Although the PRVs became the de facto government standards, their social credibility was tenuous from the beginning. Many citizens felt that they were too lax. While they were comparable to or stricter than standards in the United States and EU (table 1.1), critics pointed out that some of the standards were less strict than the WHO recommendations; for example, for tap water, the PRVs set 200 Bq/kg as the upper limit, while WHO's recommendation is 10 Bq/kg. Nonprofit organizations reported that some countries affected by Chernobyl had adopted even stricter standards, such as Ukraine's cesium 137 standard for drinking water of 2 Bq/L, and Belarus's of 10 Bq/L for drinking water and 100 Bq/L for dairy products (Foodwatch 2011). Some experts also called for stricter values; for instance, a professor of medicine, Nagayama Junya, at Kyusyu University proposed that cesium standards should be set at 20 Bq/kg for milk and other dairy products and 50 Bq/kg for vegetables ("Prof. Nagayama of Kyusyu University" 2012). That some foods consumed in large quantities by Japanese—fish and rice, for instance—did not have lower PRVs was also criticized.[3] Nonetheless, until the official standards were adopted in April 2012, the government screened food according to the PRVs, possibly underplaying the extent of contamination.[4]

Like Kobayashi-san, many citizens became highly concerned about the possibility of contaminated food. A number of consumer surveys show that Kobayashi-san was not an anomaly in worrying about and changing her food purchasing patterns after the accident. For instance, a survey by the Federation of Consumer Cooperatives in July 2011 found a large percentage of consumers (42 percent) trying to avoid food from the affected areas (Seko 2012). Similarly, in a government consumer survey in 2013, more than 60 percent of respondents said they cared about the place of origin of the food they buy, and of that group, 41 percent attributed their concern to fears about radiation; 19 percent responded that they would hesitate to buy Fukushima produce; and 15 percent said

Table 1.1 Comparison of Food Radiation Standards (Bq/kg)

	Drinking water	Milk	Regular foods
Japan (provisional)	200	200	500
Japan (April 2012)	10	50	100
US	1,200	1,200	1,200
EU	1,000	1,000	1,250

Source: Reconstruction Agency. 2014. *Hōshasen risuku ni kansuru kisoteki jōhō* [Basic information on radiation]. http://www.reconstruction.go.jp/topics/main-cat1/sub-cat1-1/20140218_basic_information_all.pdf.

the same about produce from Fukushima, Miyagi, and Iwate Prefectures (Consumer Affairs Agency 2013).[5]

Consumers also changed not only what they bought but also where they bought it. Like Kobayashi-san, who decided to buy more imported foods at Costco and gave up on the idea of local food, many consumers in the northern and northeastern parts of Japan began to avoid buying locally, turning away from the food localism that had been popular before the accident (Kimura and Nishiyama 2008). Farmers' markets were hit particularly hard in these areas. For instance, one study of farmers' markets in Fukushima found that they experienced a significant decline in sales (Endo and Matsumoto 2012). Farmers' markets in Miyagi Prefecture similarly suffered from a decline in the number of customers and the volume of sales (Miyagi Prefecture Division of Agriculture, Forestry, and Fisheries 2012).

Consumer avoidance of foods from the affected areas had significant impacts on prices. While the decline in sales of foods from the affected areas can be partly attributed to the decrease in the overall prefectural population, the decline in demand was a national trend, not limited to the affected areas.[6] For instance, Fukushima was famous for its peaches and sold them nationwide, but Fukushima peaches after the accident were priced 20 percent lower than the national average (Cabinet Office 2014a). From 2009 to 2012, the average price of Fukushima vegetables on the national wholesale market decreased by 18.7 percent, a much larger decline than the national average (0.2 percent) (Bank of Japan 2013). The price decline was not limited to Fukushima and impacted farmers in neighboring prefectures. Farmers in Miyagi Prefecture, for instance, reported lower prices for their produce (Miyagi Prefecture Division of Agriculture, Forestry, and Fisheries 2012). Food producers from the eastern and northeastern prefectures suffered significantly from the damage to their products' reputations after the Fukushima accident.

Fūhyōhigai: Censoring Concerned Women

Fūhyōhigai became an overarching concept that was frequently used to describe the mechanism of the decline in popularity of foods from affected areas. After the accident, fūhyōhigai specifically referred to the sales declines from concerns related to radiation contamination. It became one of the major economic concerns of the government, as it was estimated to have caused tremendous economic damage—a government estimate put fūhyōhigai damages at $13 billion in 2011 alone (Office of the Prime Minister 2011).

The concept of fūhyōhigai was useful to producers because it included a range of damages caused by the accident but otherwise not recognized. When food was found to be contaminated according to government standards and hence banned from sale by government orders, the producers could be compensated for the loss. But even when the food was not officially contaminated, consumer avoidance resulted in the loss of sales. This was the scenario in which the concept of fūhyōhigai was helpful to food producers because it allowed them to claim the reduction in sales as accident derived.

Besides this legal function, which was undoubtedly important and useful, the concept of fūhyōhigai had complex social functions as a mechanism of food policing. According to professor of communications Sekiya Naoya, the term was originally coined in the 1980s to characterize a decline in sales of seafood due to nuclear reactor accidents. Its use became commonplace to describe various cases of consumer avoidance, such as of beef after the bovine spongiform encephalopathy scandal and of spinach due to dioxin from incinerators (Sekiya 2003). Fūhyōhigai is a morally charged concept that redefines what might be simply described as changes in consumer preferences as regrettable misbehavior based on false rumors. In a context of scientific uncertainty, fūhyōhigai is a powerful tool to demarcate certain views as rumor while legitimizing others as fact. After the Fukushima accident, the concept was used to describe people who avoided foods from affected areas as fearmongers who caused much suffering to the food producers.

Fūhyōhigai crystallizes the combined power of scientism, neoliberalism, and gender, the three social forces I discussed in the introduction. Fūhyōhigai privileges science as the arbiter of truth and presents it as uncontested and unambiguous, while addressing neoliberal concerns about economic vitality. Furthermore, as I describe below in detail, post-Fukushima fūhyōhigai particularly targeted women as dangerously irrational.

For the readers of this book outside of Japan, it might be difficult to imagine how widespread and harsh the fūhyōhigai discourse was against those who expressed concerns about radiation. A good illustration might be the case of *Oishinbo* and how it became a national scandal. *Oishinbo*, a comic series widely popular since the 1980s, centers on a gourmand's quest for delicacies. In April 2014, the comic had a story where the main protagonist and his father had nasal bleeding after coming back from Fukushima, which was attributed to radiation exposure. This story caused a huge national scandal that was framed as a problematic case of fūhyōhigai, making the comic a target of strong criticism from the media, the government, and scientists. Various government institutions, including the Ministry of Environment and the Fukushima prefectural government, went so far as to issue statements criticizing *Oishinbo*. High-ranking politicians such as the mayor of Fukushima City, the secretary of the Reconstruction Agency, and the governor of Fukushima Prefecture made media appearances criticizing the comic as fūhyōhigai ("*Oishinbo* Hyōgen Ni Zannen" 2014). A professor from Fukushima University was quoted in the comic as saying, "I do not think it is possible to decontaminate the large area of Fukushima so as to enable people to live there"; he was reprimanded by the university, whose president said he "should be aware of his position as a university professor" and "refrain from spreading fūhyōhigai" ("*Oishinbo* Hamonhirogaru" 2014).[7] Joining the *Oishinbo*-bashing was Prime Minister Abe Shinzo, who, speaking of the comic, said, "the government needs to tackle baseless fūhyō[higai]" ("Abe Shushō Konkyo" 2014). In response, some people in the affected areas said that they did actually suffer from various health symptoms including nasal bleeding ("*Oishinbo* Hanadi Konkyoaru Senmonkara Hanronkaiken" 2014), but these rebuttals were brushed aside as simply nonscientific anecdotes. There might have been little scientific proof that radiation at the Fukushima level would cause nasal bleeding, but the politically charged responses to the comic reflect the pervasive and harsh censoring of radiation concerns in the name of fūhyōhigai.

Fūhyōhigai criticism implicitly (and sometimes explicitly) targeted women. In general, women were found to be more concerned about food safety. For instance, a 2012 survey of consumers by the government showed that while radiation contamination was the biggest concern related to food safety for both men and women, 87.6 percent of women in comparison with 68.9 percent of men expressed this concern. Moreover, a higher percentage of women than men said they changed their food purchasing patterns (Food Safety Commission 2012).[8] The stronger concerns of women about radiation contamination of food are related to a broader concern and wariness about nuclear energy historically found among more women than men. In Japan and other advanced capitalist societies, studies of people's attitudes toward radiation risks have usually found that women are more concerned about radiation contamination and its health impacts than men (Flynn, Slovic, and Mertz 1994; Watanuki 1987).[9]

Women were also seen as culpable, as they were the ones who shouldered most food-related tasks in households. While the professional culinary scene is dominated by men, domestic food tasks are done primarily by women in Japan (Holthus and Tanaka 2013). Shopping for ingredients and cooking food at home are mostly women's jobs in Japan, which makes their role highly visible in food-related scandals.

The explicit chiding of women as responsible for fūhyōhigai was often linked with their perceived weakness in technoscientific matters. For instance, Matsunaga Kazuki, the author of *Food Safety for Mothers*, was critical of the consumer reaction to radioactive contamination, which she said was unnecessary because the government had institutionalized "constant monitoring tests" that obtained "the result of non detectable (N.D.) in the vast majority of tests" (Matsunaga 2011a). In her portrayal, irrational consumer panic after the accident was caused by women who acted out of ignorance about food safety risks. As she wrote, "After the Fukushima No. 1 reactor accident, it was women, particularly mothers, who were concerned *and confused* about food contamination" (Matsunaga 2012, emphasis added). Matsunaga was not alone in criticizing mothers for acting irrationally. A professor of nutrition at Gunma University,

Takahashi Kuniko, criticized fūhyōhigai and linked it to what she described as an unfortunate "women's propensity to food faddism" (Takahashi K. 2012).

Such sanctioning of women echoes through the history of women's activism against contamination. As many feminist scholars have shown, information and data that are highly relevant to women's lives tend to be understudied or withheld by male-dominated expert communities (Proctor and Schiebinger 2008; Tuana 2006; Schiebinger 2007). Yet far from simply remaining victims of such ignorance and uncertainty, women have worked to overcome it again and again. For instance, the women's health movement has pressured the medical community to conduct more clinical studies specifically on women's health issues in the United States (Morgen 2002). The women in Love Canal, near Buffalo, New York, collected data on childhood leukemia and other illnesses in their neighborhoods and found significantly high local rates of morbidity and mortality, successfully confronting the government authorities with their findings (Blum 2008). These women's actions met harsh criticism for being irrational and unscientific. Women in Love Canal, for instance, were condemned for hampering the community's economic development and lowering the prices of real estate by what many saw as an unfounded accusation of contamination (Gibbs and Levine 1982). Environmental activist women are commonly characterized as "hysterical housewives," reflecting the "sexist policing" (Seager 1996, 279) of a patriarchal society that tries to keep them silent.

The sexist policing that took place after the Fukushima accident in the name of preventing fūhyōhigai was widespread, going beyond the statements issued by experts and government officials. On the Internet, particularly Twitter, people who were concerned about radiation were ridiculed as having a hōsha-nō (radiation brain), a pun on hōshanō (radiation) and nō (brain) ("Hōshanō Towa" 2011). A closely related term was explicit in its gendered connotation: nō-mama (radiation brain moms) were mothers with radiation brain. Reflecting a widespread understanding of maternal overreaction, mothers who raised concerns about radiation contamination were chastised as having a different kind of brain, one that was unscientific and unthinking.

Furthermore, the notion of fūhyōhigai encompassed a broad range of things, categorically describing them as baseless rumors about and discrimination against the affected areas. Prejudice against people from

Fukushima such as refusal to admit evacuees to schools and bullying was also described as fūhyōhigai ("Fukushimakarano Hinansha" 2012). Once it was categorically described as fūhyōhigai, mothers' avoidance of food from contaminated areas became a similar kind of discriminatory action against people from the affected areas.

In the characterization of both food avoidance and acts of discrimination against individuals as instances of fūhyōhigai, the profound difference between them was obfuscated—without rigorous testing of food, there remained the possibility of actual contamination. Note that there were few means for women to make sure that they were avoiding contaminated food for months after the accident. Few places offered testing services for regular citizens. Citizens could bring food to private laboratories and testing institutions, but the cost of testing tended to be high, sometimes running over $50 per sample, and it was impossible to test every item fed to a family. Access to testing facilities was an unmet need that resulted in a subsequent wave of citizen radiation-measuring organizations being established (see chapter 4). Except for rice from Fukushima, of which the entire harvest has been tested since fall 2011, only samples are tested by the government. That the lowest detectable level of the government tests tended to be high and that contamination levels varied widely even within the same district were sources of concern to many consumers. Furthermore, as the decontamination work continues to release radioactive cesium into the environment, scientific predictions of the movement of radioactive cesium were not warranted.[10] But the broad brush strokes of fūhyōhigai painted consumer food avoidance as the same kind of prejudiced and disgraceful actions that kept refugee children from attending school.

Choice of food—including the decision to eat or not to eat food from the affected areas—could be considered an individual decision to be respected, but fūhyōhigai ascribed a sense of heroism and pride to the former (eating), and embarrassment and shame to the latter (not eating). Indeed, the particularly powerful function of fūhyōhigai discourse was to create feelings of guilt and shame. Women who avoided food from the affected areas were construed as causing pain and suffering to people in the affected areas. The fūhyōhigai discourse effectively deflected culpability away from the nuclear reactors' operator, TEPCO, and the government and onto ordinary women. It framed the suffering of farmers and fishermen as caused more by consumer panic than by the nuclear accident itself.[11]

The fūhyōhigai sanctions against mothers are highly contradictory, as the preparation of good food is usually integral to the Japanese understanding of proper motherhood. In Japan, food is entangled in an ideology of motherhood that demands cooking as a core requirement of being a good mother. Historically, motherhood was linked to the notion of nation building through the Meiji-era concept of *ryōsai kenbo* (good wife wise mother), which guided Japanese women to support the *ie* (household) as the critical unit of the empire of Japan. Today, the mother as a modern imperial subject has been replaced with the tender image of the *yasashii okāsan*, the gentle mother. The gentle mothers are no less subject to pressure to perform good mothering. The postwar economic boom created a new class of full-time stay-at-home wives (*shufu*) whose job was to be professional mothers. Their duties were to look after household chores while their husbands were largely absent from the home as corporate "worker bees" and to devote themselves to child rearing to prepare their children for the tough academic competition of a society built on a hierarchy of educational attainment (Holloway 2010; Borovoy 2005).

These gentle mothers who anchor Japanese familial life are also expected to provide good food. Mother's food—or "mother's taste" (*ofukuro no aji*)—is a symbol of good food, filled with the sense of affection and nostalgia. Since the 1990s, with growing concern over the rise in obesity and chronic diseases, mother's food is increasingly featured as the foundation for a healthy and productive nation as well (Kimura 2011). In response to concerns about diet-related health problems and the deterioration of healthy dietary practices among Japanese, the government launched a *shokuiku* (food education) campaign in the first decade of the 2000s. In addition to health benefits, it emphasized the moral value of home-cooked meals, not only as an antidote to nutrition-poor fast-food and take-out meals, but also as a space of moral education and discipline for children (Alexy 2011; Kimura 2013a). Mothers then were expected to provide healthy and safe food for children in support of healthy families and nationhood, but their efforts to try to meet that ideal brought them condemnation after the nuclear accident.

Historically, Japanese culture tends to place a high value on loyalty and obedience as moral attributes in order to maintain the harmony of the larger collective (Lebra 1976; Nakane 1970). Going against the government's safety pronouncements went against the value of obedience to the government. Food avoidance by women, who are traditionally placed in a socially subordinate status, appeared an even bigger transgression that disrupted the government's postdisaster plan for "the rebirth of Japan," which was to be based on "mutual help and cooperation by all Japanese nationals" (Great East Japan Earthquake Reconstruction Headquarters 2011, 3).

As Kamiyama Michiko of Food Safety Citizens' Watch, a nonprofit group, wrote in a letter to the Food Safety Commission in 2013, when there were few ways for consumers to ensure the safety of food that they ate, "avoiding buying food is not fūhyōhigai, which is presumed to be baseless, but is a right of consumers" (Kamiyama 2013). But through a mechanism of "control by controlling emotions" (Papadopoulos, Stephenson, and Tsianos 2008), mothers were shamed and reprimanded for causing pain to producers and even to their own children, and at a high cost to national unity and the economy. Riding on a cultural coding of women as emotional and weak on scientific issues, the discourse of fūhyōhigai humiliated these women for being plagued with emotion and for engaging in shameful actions. The postaccident strategies of mothers could be seen as vigilant, dutiful, and caring, but the fūhyōhigai discourse instead painted a picture of these women as thoughtless, traitorous, and discriminatory.

Uncertainty in Science and Certainty in Government Pronouncements

Did these mothers deserve to be ridiculed as radiation brain moms who did not understand the science of radiation? Was their concern about food contamination overblown? I do not intend to evaluate epidemiological and medical studies on the health impacts of internal radiation from exposure through ingested or inhaled radioactive materials. Nonetheless, it is worth noting that the science on internal radiation is riddled with disagreement even among experts. The standards that the Japanese government used to delineate dangerous from safe, contaminated from clean, were dependent upon layers of assumptions, few of which were uncontroversial.

For instance, the most comprehensive and long-term data on radiation impacts are those on atomic bomb blast survivors from Hiroshima and Nagasaki. This data set is usually considered "the epidemiological gold standard for assessing radiation health-effects in human beings" (Little et al. 2004). However, historian Takahashi Hiroko, who studies the development of radiation research in the United States and Japan, argues that the atomic bomb survivor data are seriously flawed, and historical and geopolitical issues need to be taken into consideration to evaluate them. The data are managed by a research institute in Hiroshima called Radiation Effects Research Foundation (RERF), which, although located in Japan, was established by the United States immediately after the end of World War II. Originally called the Atomic Bomb Casualty Commission (ABCC), it was created to study the impacts of the nuclear weapons used in Japan. Takahashi argues that the United States intended the ABCC/RERF to focus on external radiation, disregarding or actively stopping research on internal radiation. The US government, facing global criticism for its use of atomic bombs and also having to justify stationing its troops on Japanese soil, tried to depict the bombs as causing only immediate death by explosion but not long-term health impacts (Takahashi H. 2012, 59–64). The notion of internal radiation would contradict such a position. The United States insisted that the bombs were clean weapons, because they exploded at high altitude, diluting the effects of the fallout, and had no lingering effects after the explosion. Historian Susan Lindee similarly summarized the US attitude on internal radiation as follows: "The Americans did not include the estimates of internal radiation, that is, inhaled or ingested radioactive particles, in their calculations. Nor did they include estimates of exposure to residual radiation, even for those near the hypocenter who might have remained in the area for some time after the bombings" (2008, 28). The US position was incongruent with the notion of internal radiation that would have long-term impacts by accumulating within the body, which seems to have colored what kind of research has been done at RERF.

It has also been pointed out that RERF was shaped not only by the US intention to minimize the issue of long-term effects of radiation but also by the Japanese government's desire to reduce the number of people who were eligible for victims' health benefits. Even though nearly 300,000 people were granted Atomic Bomb Survivor's Certificates, the government recognized only 2,000 of them as atomic bomb injury victims whose medical expenses would be covered by the government and who would be eligible for special health care allowances. The government's ability to reject applications for the certificates depended on defining what counted as radiation exposure as external radiation, as well as on acknowledging only a limited range of possible health consequences of exposure.[12]

These political pressures to treat only immediate explosion impacts as atomic bomb impacts have influenced ABCC/RERF's research, as Takahashi points out: "ABCC and RERF are not systematically conducting research on internal radiation. They cannot provide 'scientific standards' on internal radiation" (Takahashi H. 2012, 290–301). There is a dearth of studies on internal radiation's health effects, as RERF itself even admits. When Okubo Toshiteru, a council member of RERF, was asked after the Fukushima accident to be the radiation advisor for Koriyama City, Fukushima, he admitted that although RERF had been studying radiation's human impacts for more than sixty years, it did not have much data on internal radiation (Morita 2012b).[13]

In the case of the Chernobyl accident, studies on health effects from internal radiation remain ambiguous. International nuclear organizations such as the International Atomic Energy Agency (IAEA) and United Nations Scientific Committee on the Effects of Atomic Radiation (UNSCEAR) insisted that Chernobyl's effect was limited. For instance, UNSCEAR's assessment of the health impacts was that apart from the dramatic increase in thyroid cancer incidence among those exposed at a young age, and some indication of an increased leukemia and cataract incidence among the workers, there is no clearly demonstrated increase in the incidence of solid cancers or leukemia due to radiation in the exposed populations. Neither is there any proof of other nonmalignant disorders that are related to ionizing radiation (UNSCEAR 2012). These international nuclear agencies claimed that psychological effects were the most significant health impacts of the accident (Morris-Suzuki 2014b).

But some studies have shown how radionuclides accumulate in the human body (Hoshi et al. 2000), and there has been an observed increase in diseases such as leukemia (Noshchenko, Bondar, and Drozdova 2010) and other, noncancerous diseases such as cataracts (Sumner 2007) and heart disease (Trivedi and Hannan 2004). It has been difficult to establish causality between internal radiation from food and specific diseases, with the possible exception of cardiovascular diseases (Bandazhevskaya et al. 2004).

In setting radiation-related standards, the Japanese government has relied upon the International Committee on Radiological Protection

(ICRP) recommendations, but their legitimacy is also highly contested. For instance, the food standard of 100 Bq/kg (for general foodstuffs) was derived from complex calculations that involve estimates of consumption volume of different categories of food, different sensitivities to exposure by age groups, and so on. Nevertheless, the Japanese government ultimately used the ICRP recommendations as the basis for radiation protection standards. Some organizations such as the European Commission of Radiological Risk criticized the ICRP's standards, arguing "that the ICRP risk coefficients are out of date and that use of these coefficients leads to radiation risks being significantly underestimated. . . . Employing the ICRP risk model to predict the health effects of radiation leads to errors which are at minimum ten fold while we are aware of studies relating to certain types of exposure that suggest that the error is even greater" (González 2012, 247). One of the points that critics raised was that the ICRP takes cancer as the biological endpoint in calculating radiation impacts, and insufficiently considers noncancer illnesses. Some studies have indicated that radiation exposure might not result in cancer deaths, but could result in cardiovascular, immune, and reproductive diseases. The ICRP does recognize the potential of noncancerous effects, but its risk coefficient does not include noncancerous impacts (see, for instance, Health Protection Agency 2009, 11).

Some also have argued that the ICRP ignores the qualitative differences between internal radiation and external radiation and that internal radiation should be considered more dangerous than external radiation, as the radioactive materials exist closer to human cells. Professor Sawada Shoji from Ryukyu University has particularly criticized the ICRP and the Japanese government for this reason. Another expert, Kodama Tatsuhiko, a medical doctor with expertise in radiation protection and a professor at the University of Tokyo, has similarly warned of the more localized and potentially stronger effects of internal radiation. In his testimony to the House of Representatives' Labor Committee on July 27, 2011, for instance, he said, "To say 'X mSv' in relation to internal radiation is meaningless. Iodine 131 accumulates in the thyroid, Thorotrast in the liver. Cesium accumulates in the urothelium and bladder" (Kodama 2011, 19). From this perspective, each radionuclide accumulates in a different part of the body and exerts differentiated and localized effects.[14]

Despite these disagreements within the scientific community, the Japanese government and international nuclear organizations portrayed a monolithic view of radiation risk and marked it as the correct and only permissible interpretation. Such a position can be seen, for instance, in a public relations video released by the government in 2012. Titled "New Standards for Radioactive Materials in Food," the video emphasized how the new standards included ample buffers and considered all age groups. Akashi Makoto of the National Institute of Radiological Sciences appeared on the show as an expert, confidently explaining, "In our daily lives, we are constantly consuming radioactive materials in our water and food. To be concerned about the intake of radioactive materials into your body is not scientifically correct" and "food below the standard [of 100 Bq/kg] is safe." And he repeated the government mantra that "there is no confirmed evidence that a level below 100 mSv causes symptoms in our bodies" (Government of Japan 2012).

Another example of the government's construction of the "correct view of radiation risk" can be seen in a newspaper advertisement placed by the government in August 2014 (Reconstruction Agency 2014). With the headline, "Have Correct Knowledge of Radiation," the ad appeared in all the major national newspapers, including *Asahi*, *Yomiuri*, *Mainichi*, *Sankei*, *Nikkei*, and two regional papers in Fukushima (Takatori 2014). It featured two male doctors, one being Nakagawa Keiichi, a professor in the Department of Radiology and the director of the Department of Palliative Medicine at University of Tokyo. The gist of his message can be gleaned from subtitles such as "Serious Misunderstanding of Radiation Impacts" and "No Increase in Cancer in Fukushima Is Expected." The ad tried to relativize the radiation risk (e.g., "having insufficient vegetables in the diet is riskier than 100–200 mSv exposure") to make the point that people were worrying too much. In words that allow no hint of uncertainty but nonetheless betray the existence of different opinions about internal and external radiation within the scientific community, Nakagawa was quoted as saying, "Although people tend to think internal radiation is more serious than external radiation, gamma rays from cesium will penetrate the body and expose the whole body evenly, so there is no difference between external and internal [exposure]." The other expert featured in the advertisement was the director of the Human Health Division of IAEA, Rethy Chhem, who was quoted as stating, with no qualifying remarks, "Unless the exposure level is extremely high, we know that there is no health impact." Again, this comment ignores the complex scientific debates on the matter. Such obfuscation of the lack of sufficient studies and concomitant fundamental uncertainty about radiation's impact has been critical to food policing since the accident.

International nuclear organizations such as ICRP, IAEA, and UNSCEAR also played a role in legitimizing the government position and lending it scientific credibility after the accident. ICRP is one of the key international nuclear organizations and describes itself on its website as "an independent, international organisation" whose members "represent the leading scientists and policy makers in the field of radiological protection." ICRP sets global benchmarks on various radiological protections. The goal of IAEA is to develop a code of practice to be incorporated into national regulations; UNSCEAR's role is gathering and interpreting data on health effects, articulating the foundations for radiation protection standards based on data from UNSCEAR and other national institutions (Hecht 2012, 186; Boudia 2007, 399). The expert members of these organizations tend to overlap significantly (Nakagawa 1991, 77–81), constituting a powerful scientific authority behind the global pronuclear regime. These organizations are part of what some observers call the international nuclear village (Japan Scientists' Association 2014).

The international nuclear village had a lot at stake in the perceptions of Fukushima. The director of IAEA, Amano Yukiya, admitted that "the Fukushima Daiichi nuclear accident damaged confidence in nuclear power," and IAEA suggested that the growth of global nuclear power would slow down due to the accident (McDonald and Rogner 2011). The call to revisit pronuclear policies became stronger in many countries, and some, such as Italy and Germany, decided to phase out nuclear energy.

These international organizations echoed and legitimized the Japanese government's assessment that health effects from the Fukushima accident were minimal. For instance, UNSCEAR, while recognizing the possibility of more thyroid cancer among children, said there would not be an increase in other cancers or birth defects despite criticisms that its report relied on data provided by the Japanese government (see, for instance, Human Rights Now 2013).[15] In addition, IAEA played a role in legitimating the Japanese government's policies. When the government tried to relax the contamination cutoff for evacuation from 1 mSv to 20 mSv/year, for instance, IAEA held a news conference essentially affirming the controversial government position ("IAEA Urges Japan to Give Public" 2013; Shirabe 2013).

While the contribution of low-dose, chronic internal radiation to mortality and morbidity may indeed turn out to be negligible, the scientific data are incomplete and contested even among the experts on the issue. The government's insistence on the certainty of the science around the health impacts of radiation exposure belies the reality of contradictory scientific findings and opinions. Sometimes, however, the lack of knowledge on internal radiation has surfaced. For instance, a member of the Food Safety Commission who headed the efforts to review the available relevant literature acknowledged that studies that focused on the effects of contaminated food were "close to nonexistent" (cited in Morita 2011) and that "impacts from low-level radiation exposure remain scientifically uncertain (given the limits of today's science)" (Yamazoe 2011, 1).[16] But the overall discourse emphasized the safety of the current situation, relegating scientific complexity to the margins.

The government's denial of uncertainty and the promulgation of one kind of correct knowledge on radiation, however, might have worked to polarize the debate, as the politicized nature of the science of radiation became increasingly clear to many citizens. Citizens understood that the academic experts were an integral part of the so-called nuclear village, which has an entrenched interest in nuclear power. Historically, Japanese public universities—among them the most prestigious universities in the country—have been considered part of the government, their faculty members civil servants. Rotating on government committees and receiving research funding from the government, many mainstream nuclear experts were thought to be prime examples of *goyōgakusha* (government-patronized scholars) who, as handmaidens of the government, were unable to speak out against the government's positions (Sugiman 2014). Their insistence on the safety of the situation therefore only helped to fuel the concerns of the many citizens who were becoming increasingly aware of the possible capture of science by the state and the industry.

Privatized Struggles and Disaster Capitalism

One of my interviewees might be called a radiation brain mom. Inoue Mika is the mother of four children; they were residing in Fukushima Prefecture when the nuclear accident happened. She did not then have much knowledge about nuclear issues, and she had not given much thought to the reactors in her prefecture before the accident. She worked for an insurance company and was busy raising her four children. On March 12, she went out to get rationed water due to the water shutdown and saw long lines in front of the gas stations, which made her realize that some people were trying to evacuate to get away from the reactors. She started paying closer attention to radiation threats. Initially skeptical of rumors about radiation, she started to doubt the government's pronouncements, particularly when it announced that it would allow 20 mSv at schools, rather than the 1 mSv standard allowed for regular citizens before the Fukushima accident. That the government could simply increase the standard—and for schoolchildren—outraged her: "I could not believe it—just like that!," Inoue-san said in the interview. At that moment, it was driven home to her that the government was not being forthcoming about what was going on and not prioritizing the health and safety of the people.

The city government's tests in summer 2011 showed that some parts of the city exceeded the level of 20 mSv per year. The results were worrisome but also showed wide variations in the contamination levels depending on locations even within the same city. Inoue-san wanted to know how bad her particular neighborhood was, and so she contacted the city office. But she could not get a solid answer to her question. She learned about citizens trying to measure radiation levels by themselves, and through them obtained a Geiger counter. When she used it, she found out that the levels both inside and outside of her house exceeded the level of the "radiation controlled area" which was the legally designated area that was off limits for regular citizens before the accident. She told me, "We were living in areas that would have been off limits except for radiation technicians before the accident." She became more worried; she stopped buying local milk and started buying more food from outside Fukushima.

She did so quietly, not talking about her worries to her family or her friends. Her husband was away, doing business overseas, but she lived with her in-laws. They were highly critical of her worries, saying that if the government was saying it was okay, she should not be worried. She told me that she could not say much after once hearing such comments from them, as she was afraid to cause further tensions among family members. Even her children—particularly the oldest—said that she worried too much. Teachers and school administrators seemed to emphasize that the impact of the accident was minimal, and everything was fine in her area. Therefore, her struggles to feed safe food to her family after the accident became a highly private, even hushed activity. Food policing worked, to use Inoue-san's own analogy, like the *jishuku* (self-imposed restraint) mood when Emperor Hirohito was dying in the late 1980s. At that time, people's awareness and fear of potential criticism for being disrespectful resulted in the voluntary cancellation or the postponement of sports and cultural events and the weddings of celebrities. Similarly, because everyone well knew the potential of being criticized for fūhyōhigai, many self-censored, policing their own behavior to act as if nothing had happened. Silence was not imposed by an iron fist of government, but rather wrapped around people like soft velvet, gently making women feel that they had to be silent.

Inoue developed a kind of strategy for finding others like herself who were similarly worried about contamination amid the façade of normality. "Most people lived as if nothing happened, so I did not want to bring it up in conversation, but sometimes I would guess, 'she is having her kids wear masks—so perhaps she is also worried,'" she said in the interview. In 2013, *Aera* magazine published a story featuring women with similar experiences, in which a woman was quoted as saying that she felt like an underground Christian during the Edo era, when they had to deny their faith by setting a foot (considered dirty) on an image of Jesus ("Marudekakurekirishitan?" 2013). To be revealed as a radiation brain mom was like being denounced as a heretic.

The Fukushima accident spawned a new market, with corporations offering solutions to mothers concerned about radiation contamination in food. When the fear of being criticized for fūhyōhigai forced many women to refrain from sharing their concerns and collectively mobilizing to demand better policies, comfort and relief often came from services and products that purportedly addressed safety concerns. Maternal distress was refashioned into the "consumer needs" on which astute corporations capitalize. The market for "becquerel-free food"—a term referring to food free of radiation contamination—was born.

As Naomi Klein (2005, 2007) observed in the US contexts of 9/11 and Hurricane Katrina, disasters often yield profitable opportunities for the private sector in a capitalist society. The triple disasters in Japan in 2011 similarly saw the private sector expanding its influence in the name of reconstruction and recovery. The economic damages of the disasters were certainly enormous, but the reconstruction projects resulted in a significant economic boom for certain industries. Construction and nuclear industries captured billions of dollars spent by the government for the work of decontamination and reconstruction. While less obvious in comparison to the windfall enjoyed by these industries, the benefits to some in the food industry are noteworthy. Food became an arena in which astute corporations could turn disaster into profit and marketing advantages. Various kinds of businesses, from retail to restaurants, began to build unique niche markets founded on radiation concerns. Women struggling to respond to radiation threats in the context of food policing often, ironically, got a helping hand from corporations.

As feminist scholars have discussed, many women feel compelled to attempt the impossible task of being a perfect mother, and capitalism, as well as science, has often extended a helping hand to women struggling to fulfill this ideal. In capitalist systems, maternal anxiety creates a profitable market for certain services and products. For instance, worries about the quality and quantity of breast milk have resulted in tremendous growth in the formula industry worldwide (Apple 1996; Kimura 2008, 2013a). Parents are now a profitable target market in publishing, with a rich variety of manuals and self-help books on effective child rearing penned every year.

After the accident, the major supermarket chains initially struggled to cope with radiation contamination, but some of them quickly learned to use it as a marketing opportunity. One strategy was to adopt radiation standards stricter than the government ones, which were criticized as too lax by many consumers. The supermarket giant Aeon, with more than a thousand stores nationwide, decided to set its own "Aeon standards" in 2011. In defiance of the government's standards, which were 500 Bq/kg (for general foodstuffs) at the time, Aeon said that they would not allow more than 50 Bq/kg for any product. Furthermore, in November 2011, the company announced that it would aim for "zero tolerance" and would publicize its own testing results on its website (Aeon Co. 2011). It is interesting that, despite the fanfare, Aeon did not screen all products. While all the beef it sold was tested following a discovery of contaminated beef in the summer of 2011, testing of other products was quite limited.[17] Nonetheless, Aeon tested a broader range of products than its competitors, and this fact was widely reported in the media. For instance, another national supermarket chain, Itō-Yōkadō, only tested its private brands of rice, vegetables, and fruits (Kanda, Nagai, and Shinohara 2011).[18] Radiation contamination provided Aeon an opportunity to establish an image of its supermarkets as stores with higher-quality food than competing supermarket chains.

The restaurant industry also responded to the nuclear accident. Places like Restaurant Non-Becquerel emerged, and some restaurants started offering special menus such as "becquerel-free lunch" and "becquerel-free kids' menu." The becquerel is the unit of measure for radioactivity, and "becquerel-free" food meant noncontaminated food. Some restaurants formed the Food Business Safety Network and promised to serve only becquerel-free food.[19] These restaurants tended to be small, independent ones, but some major players also touted stricter radiation standards. For instance, the restaurant company Zensho, which owned Sukiya, a popular restaurant chain with more than 1,900 outlets nationwide, declared in 2011 that it would screen rice, beef, and vegetables regardless of their place of origin (Zensho Co. n.d.). This might have been a strategy to differentiate itself from its competitor Yoshinoya. The latter was famous for the same kind of beef rice bowls but admitted that it was not testing its ingredients even after the cesium beef scandal.

Various recipe books were published as well, including *Japanese Food Will Save You: The Key to Radioactive Detoxing Lies in Japanese Food* (Kirasienne Shuppan 2011), *Don't Succumb to Radiation! Eighty-Eight Macrobiotic Recipes* (Okubo 2011), and *Detoxing Radiation: The Power of Japanese Food: Brown Rice, Miso and Seaweed Recipes* (Shufuno Tomo 2011). These books tended to build on the existing image of traditional Japanese food as health food, portraying, for instance, *miso* (fermented soybean paste), *umeboshi* (pickled plum), and *nattō* (fermented soybean) as counterradiation foods. The overall recommendations in these recipes usually echoed common ideas about healthy food in the contemporary Japanese context—traditional Japanese food centered around rice and vegetables with an added emphasis on fermented and seaweed products. These recipes for making becquerel-free and antiradiation food were rarely based on scientific evidence that would meet the criteria of experts, but nonetheless met the desperate need felt by many women to do something to manage the situation.

The accident also resulted in the proliferation of antiradiation products for sale. Various products were marketed as having detoxing effects. For instance, a type of nutrition supplement called Vitapecto (apple pectin) was said to detoxify the body, and it sold for about $30 for a seven-day supply. Supplements based on spirulina, a type of algae, were also said to have a good antiradiation effect, as were products with EMs, a type of microorganisms originally developed for organic farming but now used for different purposes, including drinks and food (Matsunaga 2011b).

Producers of some specific food items also claimed that their products had antiradiation power. As mentioned above, miso is a part of the traditional Japanese diet that became popular for having antiradiation efficacy. Miso manufacturers did not miss this opportunity to market their product's potency for combating internal radiation. A national manufacturer, Takeya Miso, touted the decontaminating properties of miso on its website, with a page titled "Thanks to Miso, Radiation Exposure Effect Was Mitigated" (Takeya Miso Co. n.d.). Another, smaller manufacturer, Ishii Miso, also used its website to cite experimental studies on miso's positive effects in relation to radiation. It even held a public seminar on miso's health efficacy, featuring a talk by a medical doctor titled "Radiation Protective and Anti–High Blood Pressure Properties of Miso" (Ishii Miso Co. n.d.). Despite criticism of these marketing campaigns for lacking good scientific evidence—for instance, their critics argued that they cited studies with methodological limitations and others that extrapolated from results found with animals to humans (Matsunaga 2011b)—the corporations continued to portray miso as a potent antiradiation food in their marketing efforts.

The profitable effects of such corporate opportunism might suggest that Japanese consumers were gullible and easily manipulated, but we have to situate such products' appeal to consumers in a broader landscape of Japanese corporate responses. Companies that offered safer products seemed like heroic mavericks in an environment in which the great majority of corporations leaned the opposite way—doing little to ascertain food safety and continuing to conduct business as usual. The unresponsiveness of corporations that danced to the government's tune fueled consumer concerns and made alternative products attractive in the eyes of many.

Many citizens suspected that the corporate inertia that kept companies from responding to contamination resulted in wide circulation of contaminated food on the market, and occasional media and NGO reports seemed to confirm their fears. For instance, nonprofit organizations such as Greenpeace Japan repeatedly conducted random sampling of food products from supermarket shelves and reported that many of them were contaminated. In May 2013, for example, Greenpeace Japan found that fish sold at a national supermarket chain had cesium levels of around 5–7 Bq/kg. Of the thirteen times that they conducted this kind of testing of supermarket fish products, they failed to find contaminated food only once (Greenpeace Japan 2013). This is not to say that they exceeded the government standard for fish products (100 Bq/kg), which they were well below. But many consumers felt that food contamination was inevitable due to government and corporate inaction, and that safe food could only be ensured by specific efforts on the part of individuals.

Reports of deliberate deception by corporations also seemed to confirm consumer concerns about the food on the market. As the price of produce from affected areas became significantly lower, some corporations tried to profit from the situation by selling or using such food while masking its place of origin. For instance, journalist Azuma Hirokatsu reported in December 2011 that wholesalers were falsely labeling Fukushima rice as coming from elsewhere. He observed that used rice bags with non-Fukushima labels were being sold in Fukushima, presumably to package Fukushima rice and sell it as non-Fukushima rice. Furthermore, he pointed out that a complicated system of labeling and merchandising made it difficult to trace food origins clearly. He quoted a rice retailer as saying, "Fukushima rice can be labeled as 'domestic rice' just by mixing it with other rice, and if you mix Fukushima Koshihikari variety with Hitomebore variety, that makes it a 'multivariety' rice with no indication that it came from Fukushima. It then will go to the restaurant industry. And this rice can also be used for processed foods, such as sake, sweets, rice crackers, and rice flour bread" (Azuma 2011).

This situation of deception and inaction by many corporations inevitably made some consumers highly skeptical of the safety of the food generally available on the market. With government testing insufficient, and the food industry echoing the government rhetoric that food safety was under control, consumers were left to devise their own strategies, to which some corporations catered very well. It was this context that made the corporate provision of becquerel-free, detoxing food attractive to many consumers.

Yet another difficulty for consumers was that even safe products might not be what the corporations portrayed them to be. The claims that certain foods had antiradiation properties were rarely rooted in solid scientific studies. The claims of rigorous screening also sometimes turned out to be misleading. For instance, one of the mail-order vegetable companies touted the strictness of its radiation standards and testing. However, it was subsequently reported that the company tested its samples for less than twenty minutes, although the type of detector it was using would have required a much longer time to reach the level of precision it was advertising. The company had marketed a product line called Babies and Kids vegetable boxes, which it claimed were under 5–10 Bq/kg, and this was one of the reasons why its membership grew rapidly after the accident. Yet despite the proclaimed safety of its products, a significant doubt was raised that the company was doing what it said it was doing to ensure the safety of its food (Satō and Yamane 2012).

The Fukushima accident forced women to act as vigilantes to protect themselves, their children, and their other family members from harmful substances (Holdgrun and Holthus 2014). But necessary information was not forthcoming from the government or related scientific experts. The government data on food contamination came slowly and sporadically; the government standards for screening food were seen by many as too lax; and many affiliated scientists emphasized the safety of food. In the midst of confusing claims and counterclaims on the extent of food contamination and denial and assurances from government officials and pronuclear experts, desperate mothers had to devise various strategies to find safer food and ways to decontaminate; avoiding produce from particular areas, changing the retailers they used, and learning to change the way they cooked. This was done mostly without guidance from the government or scientific experts. There was little official instruction on what to eat, what not to eat, or how to cook after the nuclear accident. Rather, officials underplayed the risk and advised against mothers doing anything out of the ordinary.

The profound irony for consumers was that capitalism worked not only to offer possible solutions to the problem of contamination—if one hand of capitalism offered detoxing products and safe produce, the other hand compounded the problem by masking contamination and falsifying labels. Whether highlighting or underplaying radiation threats, corporations turned out to be unstable and insufficiently trustworthy partners for concerned women. While both contamination and consumer concern about it could be profitable in the postdisaster capitalist economy, uncertainty only grew for consumers.

Conclusion: Class Stratification of
Access to Becquerel-Free Food

The way that becquerel-free food and detoxing food became commodified raises the question of class stratification of safe food after the nuclear disaster. The troubling impacts of commodification of food safety hit home when I read a long essay written by Nitta Ikuko, a single mother of three young children in Kawamata, Fukushima Prefecture (Nitta 2012). I found her essay in an obscure magazine called *Musubu* that gives regular citizens an opportunity for their voices to be heard on various social issues in Japan. Let me summarize her story here.

Immediately after the accident, Nitta fled Fukushima, evacuating to Wakayama Prefecture with her children. She went back to her home in Kawamata a month later to bring back some of her family's possessions. As she was a single mother with a meager wage, she could not afford to throw out many things, and the evacuation had already been costly. Among the things that she packed in her car was a bag of rice left in the kitchen.

Upon returning to Wakayama Prefecture, she started to use that rice, and she noticed horrible things happening. Strange health issues emerged—rashes, cracked skin, and stomachaches. Her throat felt like it was burning after eating the rice. She writes about her enormous regret: "I learned from a website that many people were experiencing similar symptoms. I had diarrhea, and my children were not doing well either—they had itchy eyes, runny noses, and stomach pains. For the first time it hit me that it might be because of internal radiation" (Nitta 2012, 27). She and her kids felt much better after throwing out the bag. Nitta blamed herself for maternal neglect; she writes, "I thought I was wise because we evacuated at an early stage in the crisis, but what a foolish mother I was. And there is no mending internal radiation. I cannot apologize enough to my children. I cannot regret enough. I told my children honestly and apologized. They were surprised but immediately told me, 'Mother, it is okay. Don't worry. We are fine.' Their gentleness made me cry. Although they accepted my apology, I cannot erase the fact that I exposed them to radiation" (27).

Government and scientific experts largely failed to offer practical advice such as telling mothers like Nitta not to eat the food left in the evacuation zone. And it was not until much later that they started offering voluntary evacuees like Nitta material and financial help, which might have eased the financial pressure that made that bag of rice seem worth saving.

That Nitta was a single mother is no coincidence, as the ability to be a good mother has always been highly class stratified. The basic understanding of a good mother in Japan has historically assumed a certain class status. While it may not be explicitly stated, ideal motherhood is clearly the province of full-time homemakers, the assumption being that they are married to a salaried man with a stable income, despite the contemporary reality that such women are increasingly rare due to the collapse of the lifetime employment system and corporate paternalism since the 1990s. In addition, the growing commodification of motherhood through various corporate services and products further segregates mothers who can afford to be "good" and those who cannot.

When the uncertainty of scientific knowledge on internal radiation was concealed and citizens' concerns were chastised as foolish and dangerous, a helping hand for the inhabitants of the contaminated landscape came not from the government, TEPCO, or affiliated experts, but from private industry. There emerged an industry that catered to the unsatisfied maternal needs for *anshin* (peace of mind) about the quality of food. While their services and products were often appreciated by mothers, the privatization of food safety in this way has serious implications for equity and justice, as it further stratified access to safe food by socioeconomic status. Mothers of higher socioeconomic status could afford to buy mail-order food from unaffected places; to shop at stores that stocked exclusively non-Fukushima produce; and to eat out at the "safety network" restaurants that conducted vigorous radiation testing of their ingredients. The class stratification of access to good food is already widespread in the food system in general, not just access to becquerel-free food. High-quality food—such as organic, locally grown, fair-trade food—is often sold at a market premium at high-end grocery stores. The quest for safe and good food in the neoliberal economy tends to be refashioned into a "yuppie" pursuit of the wealthy (Guthman 2003).

It is in the patriarchal, scientized, and class-segregated structure of motherhood in Japan that Japanese women's struggles with contaminated food ought to be situated. Those without time and resources to spare had to live with lingering fear and the guilt of not being a good mother, and had to make an extra effort to try to provide safe food for their families and themselves.

TWO

Engineering Citizens

Sociologist Ulrich Beck (1992) described modern society as a risk society where distribution of risk, rather than wealth, is at the heart of social controversies. If risk is the defining feature of our time, it is perhaps not a surprise that *risk communication* has come to be a key term in food politics as well. As various food-related risks have stirred social controversies—think genetically modified organisms, pesticide residues, food additives, growth hormones in milk, and so on—the ensuing policy debates have tended to conclude with a call for better risk communication in addition to risk assessment and risk control.

An official definition of risk communication is "mutual exchange of opinions among stakeholders in assessing and controlling risks" (Tokuda 2003, 3). While it may nod to interactive decision making and stakeholder involvement, in practice, risk communication often assumes a knowledge deficiency model in which it is the public's scientific illiteracy that causes controversies. In food politics, the implicit assumption is too frequently that if only the public understood science better, the food-related controversy of the day would be resolved. Risk communication can be a way to spread an officially sanctioned interpretation of risk couched in science-based and neutral-seeming words.

The Fukushima nuclear accident prompted a proliferation of risk communication-qua-information control. Seeing the rise in public concern, Japanese government officials and scientists repeatedly emphasized the need for better risk communication. But risk communication in this context shied away from opening up debate and airing multiple viewpoints and interpretations of radiation risks and veered toward a kind of marketing of government-sanctioned messages. Indeed, the government considered risk communication after the nuclear disaster as a tool to counter fūhyōhigai (harmful rumors). As the minister of state for consumer and food affairs, Mori Masako, explained, "we are aggressively developing risk communication" as "it is important to have consumers understand that all the foods on the market are below the standards and that they are safe" (Mori 2014). Consumers acting as if they did not believe that food was safe were considered to be guilty of fūhyōhigai, and risk communication would rectify their misunderstandings. Post-Fukushima risk communication by the authorities was a way to guide public opinion in a particular direction and mold it into a particular shape, masquerading as a scientific literacy program.

Not assuming that citizens are so easily brainwashed, this chapter considers risk communication as a moment of neoliberal governmentality in which a particular kind of citizen-subject is enacted and reinforced. I make two important observations in regard to risk communication as a tool for food policing. First, risk communication increasingly utilizes grassroots groups and lay citizens not only as the targets of information dissemination but also as messengers who can convey information to their fellow citizens. The underlying dynamic here is that of a neoliberal partnership between the government, the corporate sector, and nonprofit organizations that together constitute the regime of government (Jessop 2002). This practice of risk management is also driven by the realization that talking to laypeople is sometimes best done by other laypeople, particularly when the distrust of scientific or governmental institutions is high—which was certainly the case after the Fukushima accident.

The second point is that risk communication increasingly deploys women as spokespeople on behalf of government authorities and scientific experts. Because women on average are considered more risk averse, more suspicious of new technologies, and more wary of potential contamination and pollutants, risk communication often targets women as a group that needs better scientific understanding (Slovic 1999). Furthermore, who better to talk to women than women themselves? Women are no longer portrayed as passive recipients of scientific wisdom; rather, they are to be actively mobilized to participate in disseminating the officially sanctioned understanding of risk.

This chapter's analysis shows that the nuclear industry has not simply manipulated gullible women into becoming its allies and speaking for its interests, however. A complex use of feminist ideas has been instrumental in creating a comfortable relationship between nuclear power and women. First, nuclear power was framed as a liberatory power, within the modernist theme of technoscience as a tool to emancipate women from drudgery. This framework—similar to the one discussed by Lin Nelson (1984) in the American context in the 1980s—positions risk as a product of the human progress that is essential for female empowerment and liberation.[1] I argue that there is another, more recent, discourse linked to what McRobbie (2009, 57) calls the "postfeminist gender settlement," which describes a contemporary gender politics in which women are considered equal with men and imbued with economic potential in an official pretense that helps to obfuscate ongoing injustice. This kind of settlement has high costs for women: Because postfeminism and neoliberalism are normalized in this discourse, criticism of existing structures of power, including patriarchy and the neoliberal economic order, becomes difficult. The nuclear industry invites women to behave as rational economic beings, as actors who realize the competitive value of nuclear power. But this is not an invitation to evaluate the overall economic regime that prioritizes economic growth and externalizes the health and environmental costs of nuclear power. If the earlier nuclear industry's use of women aligned itself with liberal feminism, the newer discourse considers women as economically astute and aspirational, encouraging them to choose nuclear power as the economically rational option, and to bravely take on its risks.

A change that brings a greater role for women in policy issues, particularly where they have been sharply underrepresented, as in technoscientific fields, seems like a wonderful feminist moment to be celebrated. This has been the framing of women as risk communicators preferred by the authorities and the nuclear industry. But I will point out that this particular role is rooted in traditional gender stereotypes, such as the view that women have a special ability to empathize and to speak with feeling. Furthermore, the postfeminist appeal to women is rooted in an implicit endorsement of neoliberalism without problematizing its impacts—female disempowerment and further marginalization of subaltern groups, including many women from the working class, minority communities, and with some forms of disability. Moreover, postfeminist femininity interpellates women as individuals requiring self-improvement, rather than supporting collective mobilization for social justice (Negra 2014). Instead of a feminist moment, the emergence of women as risk communicators for the nuclear industry should be considered a moment of feminist ideas being co-opted, in Nancy Fraser's (2013) words, as "a handmaiden of capitalism."

Food policing is not only a top-down process imposed by the powerful elites on the innocent masses. The government and the elites also cultivate the seeds of food policing among citizens, and food policing can be aligned with the feminist tropes of female empowerment and women-to-women support. In the same way that private capital often co-opts images of feminist empowerment in marketing (feminist consumerism), the nuclear technocracy has enlisted women to raise their voices insofar as they do not disturb the interests of the political, economic, and technoscientific establishment.

Radiation Risk Communicators: Teaching the Correct Way to Be Concerned

It was not a coincidence that risk communication became a slogan of food policing after the Fukushima nuclear accident. Risk communication had already become one of the important concepts in food governance in Japan in the 2000s. The discovery of mad cow disease (bovine spongiform encephalopathy) in Japan prompted the introduction of the Food Safety Basic Law in 2003, which made the language of risk central to food governance in Japan. It officially established risk analysis, risk control, and risk communication as three important pillars of food governance.

As made clear in this law's definition of risk communication as "mutual exchange of opinions among stakeholders in assessing and controlling risks" (Tokuda 2003, 3), risk communication is presumably a dialogue-oriented, two-way process. Nevertheless, the government has tended to take the view that the public's knowledge deficiency, in which lay people insufficiently understand information and science, is the central problem of risk communication. For instance, a journalist, Koide Goro, criticized the ethos of Japanese risk communication as follows: "if experts enlighten the public in a 'gentle' manner, the public will have the same opinion as them, and they will be able to 'be afraid correctly'" (Koide 2013, 436).[2] In this framework, food risk communication means the improved transmission of scientific information to laypeople, with the ultimate objective that those laypeople accept some level of risk in food as necessary and inevitable.

The Fukushima accident brought a resurgence of calls for better risk communication in food governance. For instance, a member of the government's Radiation Council and professor of medicine, Ōno Kazuko, commented, "risk communication has been relegated to each prefecture, but it is necessary to nurture human resources who could do these things. We need to invest much budget and time in food-related risk communicators in each prefecture. Otherwise, mothers and general consumers who are concerned and terrified that 1 Bq of radioactive cesium might kill them will continue to exist in Japan" (Radiation Council 2012).

Evident in this comment is not only the perceived need for risk communication (especially for mothers) but the need to do it from the bottom up. The government responded to this perceived need by starting a program to train a group of people it calls radiation risk communicators (RRC).[3] Started by the Consumer Affairs Agency in 2013, the RRC program aimed to improve risk communication in relation to radiation threats by creating a cadre of citizens who were knowledgeable about radiation risks in food. The idea was that these trained RRCs could then transmit the correct information to the general public. The scope of the project was not insignificant. It was implemented in all forty-seven prefectures, and a total of 3,366 people attended trainings in fiscal year 2013 alone; the training of an additional 2,000 people was the target for 2014.

The Consumer Affairs Agency created the training program for would-be RRCs. It consisted of several lectures by agency staff and university professors who specialized in nuclear physics or related fields, as well as the screening of a government-produced DVD on food safety and radiation. One lecture on the topic of communication skills was often given by a communications expert such as a former TV anchor. The training lasted for one or two days (depending on the availability of the speakers) and upon completion, each participant received a certificate with the stamp of the minister of the Consumer Affairs Agency.[4]

What was the correct understanding of the risk of radiation in food constructed in this program? The DVD made for the RRC program (Government of Japan 2013) is indicative of the specific direction of risk communication. The twelve-minute DVD covers basic information about radiation and government safety mechanisms, and its dry tone feels like that of general science educational materials. However, its central ethos is clear from the very beginning when the minister of consumer affairs is shown saying, "One year from the accident, radioactive materials in food are decreasing. Foods that are on the market are below the government standards." She goes on to connect consumer concerns with damage to food producers: "On the other hand, there are people who are still concerned. From the perspective of the producing regions, fūhyōhigai is far from over." Similar comments permeate the program, which is interspersed with quotations from several experts repeating that food is generally safe. Charts shown also underscore the rarity of the discovery of food exceeding the government standards. Moreover, while the Consumer Affairs Agency created this DVD, actual execution of the training programs was relegated to two outside organizations, one of which was a foundation called the Japan Atomic Energy Relations Organization, which is funded by the utility industry and nuclear power plant manufacturers and has been at the forefront of public relations campaigns on behalf of the nuclear power industry in Japan.[5]

The point of the RRC training program was not only to educate those who participated in it, but to use them as a cadre of knowledgeable citizens who could spread such information to their fellow citizens through their individual social networks. Upon finishing the training, the RRCs were given a form to use to report back to the Consumer Affairs Agency about what kind of local activities they conducted. The agency envisioned that these RRCs would hold workshops and give lectures at local venues such as schools and preschools, particularly targeting parents. It was expected that such a grassroots approach would be more effective in combating fūhyōhigai.

The use of RRCs reflects the overall trend in post-Fukushima food policing to engineer social consensus from within and from the ground up. It is through lay citizens and their networks in their communities that the official version of radiation risk interpretation is to be cultivated and spread.[6]

Neoliberal Citizens and Radiation
Culture: ETHOS Fukushima

Controversies over food risks increasingly go beyond national borders and involve various international expert organizations. Risks of all kinds are now managed by such organizations rather than within the framework of a single sovereign state (Papadopoulos, Stephenson, and Tsianos 2008). Standards and norms that become globally accepted reference points for domestic laws and regulations are thus decided from afar by international experts, with real consequences for people's lives. These global technocracies are often the source of dominant models of risk analysis and assessment. While their authority depends upon the weight of their scientific credentials, this kind of "state operating at a distance" (Swyngedouw 2010, 3) needs to consciously enhance its legitimacy as it does not have direct accountability to the people whose lives and livelihood are significantly impacted by its recommendations and norms. The post-Fukushima dynamics of risk communication reflect the transnational technocrats' need for legitimation in the mobilization of citizens in particular locales to refashion the globally sanctioned risk paradigm as consensus-based and locally desired.

Take, for instance, a project by the International Commission on Radiological Protection (ICRP) called ETHOS Fukushima. A key international nuclear organization, ICRP describes itself as "an independent, international organization" whose members "represent the leading scientists and policy makers in the field of radiological protection" (see ICRP's website at icrp.org). Established by physicists and radiologists who wanted to define limits for their own occupational exposure, it has become an organization that sets standards for radiological protection to serve as a basis for domestic regulations in various countries. The Japanese nuclear industry and government regulatory bodies have close relationships with ICRP, and Japanese domestic standards and laws have drawn heavily upon its recommendations.

After the Fukushima nuclear accident, ICRP was active in various capacities, and one of their projects was called ETHOS Fukushima. It was modeled after a series of projects with the same name (ETHOS) in the Chernobyl-affected areas a decade earlier. According to French sociologist Sezin Topçu, the original ETHOS was financed by the European Commission and managed by Mutadis, a private French consultancy firm and the French Nuclear Protection Evaluation Center (CEPN) which is an organization composed of French public utilities, Institute of Radiological Protection and Nuclear Safety, French Alternative Energies and Atomic Energy Commission, and Areva, a French nuclear reactor giant (Topçu 2013).

Central to the ETHOS project was the idea of "practical radiation protection culture" (PRPC). According to Jacques Lochard, a French economist who was involved in ETHOS and his collaborators, PRPC refers to a culture where residents engage in "self-help protective actions" by being "properly informed and ... trained (to use the means and equipment provided by the authorities) in order to take informed decisions concerning their own protection, with a net benefit" (Lochard et al. 2009, 26). ETHOS aimed to instill PRPC into residents in the contaminated areas after Chernobyl, so that thereby they could continue living in the contaminated areas rather than evacuating.

The concept of PRPC reflects two broader ideologies increasingly espoused by the international nuclear community: Individuals have the responsibility to minimize radiation harm to themselves, and a cost-benefit calculation is necessary to design protective measures. Notice the very peculiar language in Lochard's definition of PRPC, with its emphasis on the individual responsibility of residents to protect themselves ("their own protection") and its hint of the economistic valuation of protective measures ("with a net benefit"). A little historical context is useful in understanding the genealogy of PRPC. It was first proposed when the affected governments could no longer bear the costs of clean-up and evacuation after Chernobyl, and when these costs also reached the point where they would have negative impacts on the economic valuation of the nuclear power industry elsewhere (Topçu 2013). Thus PRPC was a conceptual tool to shift the responsibility for the protection of health and safety to individuals and to curb the costs of radiological protection by prioritizing continued settlement rather than evacuation.

Post-Fukushima Japan faced the mounting cost of the accident: It became increasingly clear that decontamination to the previously declared goal of less than 1 mSv/year would be extremely costly, while the cost of the evacuations already stressed the national budget. More than 150,000 Fukushima residents were still evacuated in 2014, and the government has had to inject more than $40 billion into the owner of the Fukushima reactors, Tokyo Electric Power Company (TEPCO) to keep it afloat ("Seifu Genpatsu Baisyōde" 2014).[7] The preaccident legal framework in Japan assumed 1 mSv/year as the annual dose limit for regular citizens. But as the evacuation and decontamination costs mounted, the government moved to allow more than 1 mSv and, contrary to its initial promises, started lifting evacuation orders in areas that still had higher levels of contamination. In December 2011, it reorganized zoning of the affected areas and made 20 mSv, not 1 mSv, the cutoff, rationalizing that it could be considered "safe because excess cancer risk is not scientifically recognized" under 100 mSv/year (cited in Shirabe 2013). The decision was controversial even within the government. The government committee that debated this policy had argued for 5, not 20, mSv. But 20 mSv became the allowable limit in the end. The newspaper reported that the government pushed for the higher allowance of 20 mSv, ultimately because it would ease the financial burden ("Fukushima No Kikankijyun" 2013). International actors were subsequently brought in to legitimate the government decision. In October 2013, the International Atomic Energy Agency (IAEA) sent a team of thirteen experts, who gave a news conference at which they said that the Japanese government should find an "optimal balance" between the costs and the benefits, "with a goal of achieving a dose of 20 mSv or less," mentioning 20 mSv, not 1 mSv, as the cutoff (Shirabe 2013).

Moreover, ETHOS and its cultivation of PRPC facilitated both the shift away from evacuation and the portrayal of the laxer standard as a locally desired decision. The overall message was the need for PRPC, because it could "allow inhabitants to understand and evaluate the information on the consequences of the accident and to take informed actions for reducing radiological exposure" (ICRP 2012b, 1), so that residents would choose to continue living in the contaminated areas.

On the surface, ETHOS was participatory and bottom-up, paying abundant lip service to dialogue among stakeholders, including local residents. For instance, under the ETHOS Fukushima umbrella, ICRP started holding a series of seminars called ICRP dialogue seminars and invited interested people to come and share their views.[8] In line with its self-portrayal as democratic, participatory, and citizen driven, ETHOS Fukushima particularly called for increasing participation of local residents and partnerships with nonprofit organizations. For instance, the recommendations from one dialogue seminar in Fukushima included the following: "Not-for-profit organisations (NPOs) play an important role, different from and complementary to the role of authorities, in helping communities build capacity to take effective Self-Help Protection actions" (ICRP 2012a, 2).

In fact, ETHOS found citizen partners. One example was a nonprofit organization aptly named ETHOS Fukushima. According to its website,

ETHOS Fukushima was a "Japanese ETHOS" that "aim[ed] at making it a reality for us to continue living in this wonderful Fukushima despite the nuclear disaster and to help us look to a better future" (ETHOS Fukushima n.d., 1). ETHOS Fukushima participated in multiple ICRP dialogue seminars, translated publications from the original ETHOS in Chernobyl into Japanese and posted them on its website, and visited Chernobyl-affected areas on a study tour.

Another organization in Tamura City, Fukushima Prefecture, was called the Association for Future's Creation of Tamura and Children (AFTC, Tamura to Kodomotachi no Mirai wo Kangaerukai, their translation of the name). Its leader was a middle-aged prep school teacher. In his resume, there was nothing that would suggest expertise in nuclear physics or radiation protection, but after the accident, he refashioned himself as a "radiation advisor" (although this sounds like an officially credentialed title, it is not) and started giving talks in that capacity. The city of Date even hired him for its radiation-related health consultation programs, and he gave lectures at schools on the topic. In addition to educating the public as radiation advisor and establishing AFTC, he also founded the Fukushima Stakeholder Coordinating Council (Fukushima Sutēkuhoruda Chōsei Kyōgikai) in 2012.

From his blog posts and other online materials, it is clear that his thoughts and public messages were closely aligned with those of the government and other nuclear organizations. The fact that he was invited by several international nuclear organizations including IAEA and ICRP to seminars (including ETHOS dialogue seminars) and conferences and that his organization (the Stakeholder Coordinating Council) is cochaired by Niwa Otsura of ICRP shows his close connection with the nuclear establishment. Whether his organization should be described as a pseudo-NGO fabricated by the nuclear establishment or an authentic grassroots organization, I do not have the data to answer.

Rather than speculating on his organization's authenticity, the more important point that I want to make is that these local people advocating against the evacuation, make ideal risk communicators who can be represented as the local voice. At ICRP dialogue seminars in which the aforementioned prep school teacher participated as a leader of a local nonprofit organization, he shared the story of the death of his mother, who evacuated from Fukushima to Saitama Prefecture and died there. He told this story as a parable of the cost of evacuation, saying, "Radiation is not a risk, but what is killing the elderly is evacuation and concomitant stress." His message also drew on the love of one's hometown, which was emphasized in the implicit condemnation of evacuation as abandonment of home. For instance, AFTC's website was full of passages that cry love for the homeland, such as, "We love this place Tamura, and we are proud that we live here, and we want to continue living daily lives, working, and raising children, surrounded by people we love" (Association for Future's Creation of Tamura and Children n.d.). Furthermore, the safety of continuing to live in the city was emphasized. The same website said, "There are many who are concerned about us. People outside Fukushima have invited us to evacuate there. Many have kindly offered to help the evacuation, even if only for children and pregnant women. But in relation to radiation dose level, Tamura seems safer than the central region of Fukushima. Therefore, we want to live in Tamura. Please teach us what we can do to entrust this land to our children who will bear Tamura's future." Tamura City is located close to the troubled reactors; some parts of the city are within a twelve- to eighteen-mile radius of the nuclear plant. Some areas of Tamura were still above 1 mSv/year even in 2013 (Greenpeace Japan 2013a). Some people considered it dangerous to continue living there, but the local voice represented at ETHOS forums helped justify the government decision to lift the evacuation order, framing it as a local demand and the choice of the residents. For the government and international organizations that tried to minimize the cost of the disaster response, the speaker's insistence that people just need "decontamination of minds" (*kokoro no josen*) rather than actual decontamination and evacuation was convenient and useful.

This kind of local resident is the ideal risk communicator from the perspective of ICRP, because the resident is best positioned to spread PRPC in disaster areas. The local residents are to voluntarily seek and disseminate a particular kind of mentality—PRPC—that will help local people to choose to stay there. Authorities can evade the criticism that they are abandoning their responsibilities to protect regular citizens; they can now argue that they are simply respecting the local residents' wish to live there and helping them manage individual exposure to radiation contamination.

It is impossible to completely deny that their program resonates well with local sentiment in areas where the decision to evacuate or to stay has been extremely difficult. The notion of individual choice is alluring when different interpretations exist in relation to the extent and consequences of contamination. In many parts of Fukushima, whether to evacuate, to decontaminate, and to engage in other protective actions were profoundly difficult questions for many residents. Many of them felt that they had no other option but to continue living where they were. Risk communication through presumably grassroots organizations helped to refashion such conditions as the result of their individual "choice," not as the result of the authorities' inaction and unwillingness to take responsibility in ensuring people's right to live in a clean and safe place.

Individual Responsibility and Grassroots Movements

The bottom-up, participatory approach to risk communication in nuclear power needs to be considered as part of a broader shift in thought about radiological protection in the last several decades. It is at least partially necessitated by individualization of risk in nuclear power governance.

The example of ETHOS clearly shows the implicit understanding of risk control as individual responsibility, but this individualization of risk had already begun in the nuclear industry decades earlier. The Chernobyl accident prompted the widespread use of the concept of optimization of protection, which meant the application of cost-benefit calculations in radiation protection. It was argued that the optimization of protection would be best achieved through individualized management of risk, rather than management of the whole area based on general air/soil dose levels. The rationale was that even within the same locale, individual exposure levels varied and could be lowered by cautious choices in daily lives. As a key ICRP publication emphasized, "The success of measures taken to control doses to members of the public in existing exposure situations relies heavily on the behavior of those exposed" (Lochard et al. 2009, 3).

There are serious criticisms of the individualization of radiation protection. First, the idea of optimization of protection might not necessarily result in lower exposure levels for individuals, depending on how the cost is calculated against the benefit of protective measures. As ICRP admits in one of its publications, "optimisation of protection . . . is not minimisation of dose. . . . Thus, the best option is not necessarily the one resulting in the lowest residual dose level for the individuals" (Lochard et al. 2009, 28–29). Furthermore, the assessment of radiation exposure for individuals and effectiveness of countermeasures is necessarily imprecise, making it dependent upon estimates, which are vulnerable to manipulation. The emphasis on individuals rather than the collective is also criticized for ignoring the scale of contamination, although genetic effects of radiation are more serious in a big group than a small one. Finally, the individual evaluation of risk and control might perversely promote a dilute-and-disperse approach by the authorities and the industry (Shrader-Frechette and Persson 2002). Nonetheless, individualization of protection was already becoming popular among nuclear experts by the time the Fukushima accident took place.

In order for the individualized risk approach to be ethical, it has to at least take the form of informed consent. Given the highly subjective nature of evaluating the costs and benefits of risk reduction, to meet ethical parameters, decisions need to come not from the authorities and the industry that want the minimum of protection and concomitant costs, but from people themselves. Therefore, it is not a coincidence that the international nuclear establishment now emphasizes participation by laypeople. Documents by the international nuclear aggregate are now dotted with the mention of participation and partnership with local residents.[9]

Participation, however, ought to be combined with the fostering of PRPC and a particular kind of citizen who engages in "self-help protective actions" by being "properly informed" (Lochard et al. 2009, 26). Individuals are to consider "the balance" between, "on one side, their desire to improve the situation and, on the other side, the 'burden' induced by the implementation of protective actions" (26). The role of the authorities becomes more about facilitating "processes to allow inhabitants to define, optimise, and apply their own protection strategies if required" (27), and less about minimizing the health risks and ensuring the safety of citizens.

The model of citizens here resonates strongly with the concept of the neoliberal citizen who disciplines herself to optimize her contribution and minimize her cost to the national economy. The neoliberal citizen accepts that some risk is unavoidable, engages with rational calculation of costs and benefits, and manages her own radiation exposure. Such individuation of risk calculation and the assignment of the responsibility for managing it to individuals rather than the nuclear industry and the government is an indispensable prerequisite for the touted participatory turn in risk communication.

Teaching How to Fear and How to Support Nuclear Power: Women-to-Women Communication

Risk communication by the nuclear village is not only increasingly participatory and bottom-up. Frequently, it also makes women its primary target audience and its preferred messengers. In the postaccident dynamics of risk communication, women have been recruited to do the job of teaching the right way to be concerned and to become effective ambassadors of the nuclear village.

The role of an organization called WiN (Women in Nuclear) Japan is relevant here. WiN Japan was established in 2000 and had about 250 members as of 2014. It is a national branch of a transnational organization, WiN, which was established in 1992. Its establishment was motivated by the industry's need to gain social acceptance and particularly to help reverse diminished public support after the Chernobyl accident. The industry recognized the particular importance of women; they were more likely to be opposed to nuclear power and they had already created significant antinuclear movements. As a network of female professionals in the nuclear industry, WiN aims to "promote the understanding and public awareness of the benefits of nuclear and radiation applications" (Women in Nuclear Global 2015). It now has branches across the globe, with 250,000 members in over a hundred countries.

Since its inception, WiN Japan has played an important role in cultivating women's support for nuclear energy, particularly in host communities. For instance, it has held women's meetings in the nuclear power plants' host communities in order to build favorable attitudes toward nuclear power among local residents, invited local women to nuclear power plants, and held workshops that specifically target women. WiN Japan has argued that such a "heart-to-heart" approach among women is critical to the success of the nuclear industry (Kitsunai 2006, 78).

The Fukushima nuclear disaster further strengthened the call for WiN to actively respond to the fear of radiation and the now-widespread opposition to nuclear reactors. WiN members appeared in the media after the accident to talk about the need to learn from Fukushima, but also about the importance of nuclear energy for energy security in resource-poor Japan. They also conducted community outreach targeted at women, such as a symposium involving local women in Fukushima in August 2014.

WiN Japan emphasizes the advantage of their "women's perspective" in risk communication about the nuclear disaster and nuclear energy more broadly. WiN is better equipped to convince the public than male experts because, they reason, they "think together *from women's perspective*, as we understand well why mothers might be concerned about radiation impacts on children" (quoted in Andō 2014, emphasis added). Despite their emphasis on "women's perspectives," however, the views promulgated by WiN are heavily skewed in favor of nuclear power, emphasizing the minimal risk of radiation. For instance, Ogawa Junko, the chairwoman of WiN Japan, described how she would explain food contamination to students as follows: "Your body has 7,000 Bq of radiation. . . . Even if you eat 100 Bq, the x is 7,000, so nothing to worry about" (Ogawa 2013, 16).

Nonetheless, it would be a mistake to consider WiN Japan a PR machine of the male-dominated nuclear village without at least recognizing some agency of its female members. The disaster undoubtedly produced various responses from its members, some of whom have different visions for the nuclear industry. Furthermore, it is not hard to understand how WiN members are attracted to the concept of women-to-women communication and collaboration. WiN represents women in the nuclear industry, where very few women work professionally. It provides a much-needed homosocial network for those in a male-dominated field typical in the science, technology, engineering, and mathematics-related industries.[10]

WiN Japan portrays the power of nuclear energy as linked directly and indirectly to women's liberation. The chair of WiN Japan, Ogawa Junko, said that what inspired her most when she joined WiN was a phrase that she heard at the WiN Global conference: "energy liberated women." Nuclear energy, to her, was the energy that enabled Japanese women to pursue a "happy life" different from that of "Japanese women only a hundred years ago who were occupied by household chores." She felt that nuclear energy enabled women to "make time for intellectual labor and learning" ("Ogawa Junko" n.d.). This is similar to the US nuclear industry's public relations campaigns that have portrayed nuclear-fed electricity as the source of liberation for women (Farseta 2008; Nelson 1984).

Nevertheless, WiN's apparent espousal of women's importance in the nuclear industry calls for critical evaluation from feminist perspectives. It is hard to miss the highly essentialized view of women held by WiN, which goes back to its origins. At the 1989 conference that led to WiN's inauguration, Irene Aegerter, who became its first president, called on the industry to recognize the importance of women. She said, "We know the advantages of nuclear energy to the environment. But how can we explain this to women? How can we transmit this message to women? Will they accept this message? And are they then ready to accept nuclear power?" (Aegerter 1989, 3). She then argued that the task of transmitting this message to women was best assigned to women, for two reasons. First, women are more emotional and the industry lacked the ability to convince them emotionally. Second, women's opposition stems from their inability to understand the science of nuclear energy, and the industry lacked the ability to speak to them in simple terms without jargon.[11] Women, then, hold a particularly important role in the nuclear industry because it is women who create what Aegerter called the threat of "a reign of pure emotion" (1989, 3).

Such essentialized views of women were also clear decades later, when the Fukushima accident hit. WiN Global issued a statement after the accident, relaying their sympathy to the victims and their solidarity with Japanese nuclear professionals for demonstrating how to "stay united in good and bad days and how to act in a rational manner without giving way to the emotions." It further made a resolution to "overcome the unique challenge in front of us to developing the industry" and called on WiN members to put into practice "our natural instinct to give and protect life" as women (Women in Nuclear 2011).

The example of WiN points to how the nuclear industry and expert communities have espoused a critical role for women in relaying its messages to female citizens. It was they who would cultivate the right understanding of nuclear power as beneficial and radiation risk as controllable among female citizens. While their view of women's opposition is rooted in a knowledge deficiency model that does not perceive much agency on the part of those who criticize and doubt nuclear power, the industry has skillfully employed feminist themes of emancipation and homosocial support. Using women as risk communicators, the nuclear industry has courted women's participation in the promotion of nuclear power.

Young Women as Nuclear Supporters

The nuclear village's courting of women has not been monolithic, and seems to be changing, reflecting the social environments and discourses surrounding women, particularly that of the postfeminist gender settlement. If WiN has cultivated consent to radiation risk by deploying liberal feminist language, a related yet distinctly different kind of message woos women's acceptance of nuclear power as a feminine requirement under the postfeminist gender settlement.

In an era when feminism is construed as already irrelevant, a new category of womanhood proliferates, compelling women to assume their equality with men as already achieved and aspire for material success, while at the same time pulling them away from political mobilization to challenge the largely intact patriarchy (McRobbie 2009). The postfeminist gender settlement assumes an equal playing field for women and men, and yet defines women's success as the triple achievement of beauty, motherhood, and career. Perhaps most evident in the way that Sarah Palin and Sheryl Sandberg have garnered significant female fandom as symbols of empowered women (Negra 2014), the new icon of female empowerment is a woman with material success in a corporate/entertainment world while at the same time adhering to traditional, hegemonic standards of (heterosexual) motherhood and codes of beauty. In this discourse, female empowerment comes from endless self-cultivation, in line with neoliberal aspirationalism.

The idea of postfeminism reflects a backlash against feminism; the notion that feminism is no longer necessary does not acknowledge the reality of rampant sexism and heterosexism. In Japan, the postwar decades saw a strong move toward gender equality, including institutionalization of equality in voting, employment, education, and nationality claims (Kobayashi 2004). This led to a backlash against feminism. The backlash is manifested in the growing conservative insistence on the naturalness and virtue of hegemonic femininity and masculinity as well as the value of the so-called traditional family (Wakakuwa and Fujimura-Fanselow 2011). At the same time, women's economic contributions are increasingly touted by politico-economic elites. Under neoliberalism, which followed the burst of the bubble economy and subsequent "lost decade(s)," when the Japanese economy's annual GDP growth hovered around 0.2–0.3 percent (Iwase 2013), greater female labor participation was seen as critical for national competitiveness. The shrinking population due to the sharp decline in the fertility rate also raised the stakes for convincing people to reproduce, and hence increased the cajoling of women to have more babies. The concept of the postfeminist sexual contract describes this jarring combination of cheerleading of women as economic engine and a nervous reminder about the virtues of existing sexual and social orders.

Reflecting such changes in the notion of female empowerment, the nuclear industry's message to women has also changed. Barbara Judge provides an example of such a postfeminist relationship between women and the nuclear industry and the astute cultivation of female support. Judge is a UK/US lawyer who has held important positions in the nuclear industry in Europe. Her résumé in the nuclear industry is impressive; she served as chairperson of the UK Atomic Energy Authority and was made a commander of the British Empire for her services to the nuclear industry. Already a key figure in the Euro-American nuclear industry, Judge took an increasingly visible role in Japan after the Fukushima nuclear accident. In particular, she became a deputy chair of TEPCO's Nuclear Reform Monitoring Committee, which, according to its website, is "an independent committee that conducts external monitoring and supervising" of TEPCO's reform efforts (n.d.). One of its missions is to help TEPCO improve its risk communication and Judge is in charge of it. Far from being a neutral expert on nuclear issues, Judge's views are aligned with those of TEPCO and the Japanese government. In her comment, "Approximately 20,000 lives were lost as a result of the earthquake and tsunami, but not one of those who died did so as a result of radiation. . . . Radiation experts believe that no-one will die from radiation" (Davies 2013), she seemed to minimize the severity of the accident and was evidently still committed to promoting the view of nuclear power as a safe and economical energy choice.

Judge has emphasized the importance of women for the future of nuclear power and seems to have made promoting the role of women one of her important missions in Japan. Commenting on the particular importance of herself as a part of the TEPCO team, she said, "It is often said that in every country, not just Japan, one of the groups in society that is the most against nuclear energy is women, particularly upper-middle-class women. Accordingly, I think it is important to have someone who can view and assess a safety culture from the point of view of a woman, as well as a nuclear expert" (Judge n.d.). She has consciously taken on the role of a cheerleader for women, and she presents herself as a spokesperson for women and an embodiment of female success. Touring in Japan, she underscored her struggle as a female pioneer in a male-dominated field. For instance, when she went to Fukushima as part of ICRP dialogue seminars with local residents, she highlighted the importance of female participation and said, "I was very glad to see women participated in discussion, as it is usually men who do so in Japan. Keep it up!" Defining herself as a role model for Japanese women, she went on to say, "I myself fought hard when I was young," making a "gesture of a fighting pose" as reported in the mass media (Ochi 2014). With such a narrative to encourage Japanese women to "lean in" (Sandberg 2013) to succeed like their Western sisters, she has positioned herself as a fellow fighter struggling against sexism.

But how do Japanese women view women like Judge, who are the female voices of the nuclear establishment? Between Judge and her female audience in Fukushima, a large gap exists in terms of economic means and physical mobility, despite Judge's effort to portray them as equals, or at least herself as a role model. Neoliberal aspirationalism might effectively conjure dreams and ambitions within educated upper-middle-class women, but those women who are channeled into low-wage and low-mobility sectors might not be enticed to believe that they could beat the odds and be successful like Judge. What kind of Japanese women could Judge bond with and summon as desirable female subjects of nuclear politics? The example of an organization called the Forum of Female Students for the Future of Japan opens up some understanding.[12] The forum was established in 2013 by an undergraduate student at a private university in Tokyo, as a group of female university students whose objective was to have discussions on international relations, economy, and business. Judge sits on their board.

The forum has organized multiple conferences on the theme of nuclear power and invited nuclear experts including men, but, among the experts invited, Judge seems to have made particularly strong emotional connections with the female students. An examination of the forum's Facebook posts (its primary means of communication) after seminars with Judge makes it clear that her self-conscious projection of the have-it-all woman made a strong impression on her young Japanese female audience. For young women in Japan, who are still struggling for equality with very few role models, a female figure like Judge can provide much-needed encouragement and hope. On a blog, one forum member who participated in a session with Judge wrote about how she had been struggling to figure out how to balance motherhood and career after college and how impressed she was with Judge, who seemed to have it all. She recounted how she went up to Judge after the talk and said to her in tears, "I have been at Tokyo University where more than 80% of the students are male, and I am always a minority. I have been concerned whether this was the right choice, and was agonizing over which to prioritize between motherhood and my career. I was truly moved to hear your experiences. You taught me how I could be a good mother and pursue a career. I cannot express my gratitude enough." Emphasizing her emotional connection with Judge, the young woman wrote on the blog, "Ms. Barbara held my shoulder and said 'Don't worry, you are going to be a great mother!' I cried and cried" ("Lady Barbara Judge san to no tōku sesshon" 2013). Later, she wrote about how a TEPCO representative approached her and offered her an internship.

Other comments on Judge's presentation by participants also indicate that many saw her as a female role model who had everything that is coveted under the postfeminist gender settlement—not only a successful career but physical beauty and motherhood. For instance, one participant wrote on Facebook on October 16, 2013, "I had never met anyone who achieved all in career, family, and beauty. As I listened to her, I realized that continuing to work is necessary for women to have it all. Power comes from having a career and economic capacity. Family and beauty will naturally follow career and you will become confident. Lady Barbara Judge is my female role model." That she was a mother was mentioned by several forum members, and that she was beautiful was also underscored in comments such as, "I was overwhelmed by how attractive she was. She acted gracefully and was beautiful as a woman" (Facebook, October 15, 2013).

Judge embodies the ideal woman under the postfeminist gender settlement, where female empowerment stems from the have-it-all ideal that combines financial success, heterosexual reproduction coded as "family," and physical beauty. Judge has held many powerful positions in the private and government sectors, but in line with the have-it-all ideal, she is also married and has a son. Probably in her sixties, Judge still looks youthful and always wears professional but feminine attire of jacket, skirt, and high heels, with perfectly done hair and makeup. Symbolized in her is an increasingly salient paradigm that equates female empowerment primarily with economic success achieved through individual cultivation of competence and wealth but without losing femininity, which is embodied by reproduction and beauty. McRobbie's concept of the "postfeminist masquerade" describes how such successful women's "opportunity to work and earn a living is thus offset by the emphasis on lifelong and carefully staged body maintenance as an imperative of feminine identity" (2007, 63). Aspiring young women from economically mobile families—like those in the forum who attend good universities—are particularly susceptible to such messages.

Importantly, not only the messenger (Judge) but also the message communicated to and espoused by young women in the forum bears the mark of the postfeminist gender settlement. First, women's subjecthood is construed as an economically astute, upwardly mobile one in the neoliberal world order. Women, now enlightened and empowered, are to consider nuclear power as an economically rational option, particularly in the era of global competition. Judge certainly communicated to female students that women should understand nuclear power's economic importance. This view, which apparently resonated with the forum members, portrays nuclear power as a realistic choice, and the antinuclear position as a display of naïveté based on ignorance of the realpolitik of the international economy. The neoliberal view of global economic competition undergirds the view of the economic necessity of nuclear power, in particular for Japan because it is a resource-poor country whose survival in the global market requires a reliable energy source like nuclear power. The forum's leader often emphasized her international pedigree by frequently drawing on her study abroad at Oxford University in her comments on Facebook and media interviews. The forum's implicit message to female students is that if they become more cosmopolitan and business savvy, they will understand the economic and geopolitical need for nuclear energy for Japan. Furthermore, as indicated by its name, "for the Future of Japan," the forum's viewpoint is simultaneously nationalist and internationalist. Their consideration of nuclear power is related to a nationalist calculation of economic development and global energy competition over resources. We might see the group as reflecting a recent rise in young women's conservatism in Japan, including those who participate in ultranationalist groups (Kitahara and Pak 2014; Sanami 2013). The forum's viewpoint significantly overlaps with the government's pronuclear message.[13]

While the forum's embrace of gender equality, its celebration of female role models, and its creation of a homosocial network might seem feminist, its inclination is postfeminist, to urge women to follow and mimic hegemonic economic and political logic, to be someone like Judge who has abided by the rules of the patriarchal capitalist society and is successful within those confines. The forum's motto being, "Life depends on your choice. Choice depends on your personality" (Facebook, July 20, 2013), it rarely has engaged with the question of how choice might actually be stratified by class, race, disability, citizenship, and sexual orientation. Nuclear power is embraced as the rational economic choice, but there is little in the way of sympathy for the disenfranchised, and little analysis on how the nuclear industry depends upon exploitation of the impoverished farmers and fishermen who are forced to give up or compromise their livelihood for the power plants, marginalized workers who expose themselves to radiation even in the normal operation of the power plants, and women in general who have higher health risks from radiation exposure. If being a feminist means opposing all forms of domination (not limited to sexism), the forum's call to women seems to veer toward the opposite—to help a few women to be on the side of the dominant and the powerful. Rather than seeking to challenge the dominant gender and economic orders, the forum's call to arms to (elite) women is to use it to their advantage.

Lurking behind the embrace of women as nuclear communicators are two important ideologies of our times. Postfeminism sees no need for radical collective mobilization to challenge sexism, and thus isolates sexism from other forms of oppression experienced by women. Neoliberalism selectively employs feminist themes and refashions them to fit the language of entrepreneurism and individual accountability. The neoliberal and postfeminist paradigm of female empowerment helps to frame nuclear power as a postfeminist and neoliberal choice that is just right for women.

Conclusion

The censoring of concerns about food increasingly involves NGOs, ordinary citizens, local residents, and women as key actors. Cultivating the understandings and emotions of citizens—particularly women—to mobilize support for a specific view of risk is crucial to food policing. Bottom-up and participatory risk communication makes an efficient regime of food policing, telling people how (not) to be concerned.

The participatory approach might be better than a top-down, closed-door one, and the inclusion of citizens and women satisfies a certain populism as they are portrayed as representing the popular will (Swyngedouw 2010). However, as scholars have pointed out, the nominal inclusion of "local people/residents" and "citizens" tends to become a tyrannical orthodoxy in which the power relations surrounding a project are obscured, resulting in the manufacturing of consensus within already given parameters (Cooke and Kothari 2001). Post-nuclear-accident risk communication in Japan also needs to be investigated from such a critical vantage point, and it is necessary to point out how the fragmentation of the responsibility for citizens' well-being might have driven the desire for the so-called bottom-up, participatory approach.

This chapter has shown the particular importance of women in nuclear risk communication. While it might seem to be a welcome trend from the feminist perspective, I have pointed out how the nuclear industry's embrace of women is highly influenced by gender stereotypes of women as irrational and unscientific, and in need of enlightenment and guidance. Women are considered to be useful as risk communicators because of their intrinsically feminine characteristics such as being empathetic, considerate, and emotional. Furthermore, in the neoliberal economic order, women are increasingly encouraged to choose nuclear power as an economically savvy option, ignoring the injustices rooted in nuclear power. Feminist themes have been co-opted without consideration of the intersections between sexism and other forms of oppression.

Citizens—particularly women—are no longer innocent bystanders of risk communication in nuclear politics. They are mobilized and gendered in a highly selective and peculiar manner in the governance of technoscientific risks.

THREE

School Lunches

Science, Motherhood, and Joshi Power

Every day, close to ten million students eat school lunches at public elementary and middle schools in Japan. Unlike the US school lunch program, which has often been criticized for serving unhealthy processed food, the Japanese school lunch program has generally prided itself on its quality and is officially positioned as an important and mandatory component of the curriculum by the government. Nevertheless, the government did not react promptly to the Fukushima nuclear accident to ensure the safety of school lunches. Rather, the authorities were unwilling to recognize the possibility of contamination even after contaminated vegetables were discovered several times. "There is no impact from the accident on school lunches for now," proclaimed the minister of education on March 22, 2011, trying to assuage simmering concerns among parents about radiation contamination in their children's food ("Nōsakubutsusyukkateishi" 2011).

The earliest action by the government regarding the safety of school lunches after the nuclear accident took the form of a decree from the Ministry of Education on April 5, 2011, but it was mainly concerned with the hygienic conditions of school kitchens that had been used in the emergency evacuations after the earthquake and tsunami. It made no mention of radiation contamination (Ministry of Education, Culture, Sports, Science and Technology 2011).

It took the so-called cesium beef scandal for the government to start taking concerns about school lunch contamination seriously. The cesium beef scandal started with the discovery in the summer of 2011 that beef was being sold although its contamination level exceeded the government standards (then 500 Bq/kg), with some samples as high as 2,200 Bq/kg. The subsequent investigation by the government found that at least 2,965 cattle had been fed contaminated hay before being slaughtered and sold on the market ("Hōshasenseshiumu Osengyū" 2011). Furthermore, the investigation revealed that some of the cesium beef was used for school lunches (Makishita 2013). The scandal fueled the momentum of groups in various municipalities that had already started to organize around the school lunch safety issue. In this chapter, I use the term "safe school lunch movement" to refer to these groups that were organized after the nuclear accident and analyze their strategies for mobilization. There was already a social movement centered on the quality of school lunches, which, for example, lobbied for the increased use of domestic food and opposed neoliberal restructuring. But the movement in question in this chapter was triggered by the nuclear accident, in response to which many new groups were established. The safe school lunch movement after the accident was not unified or centralized, and I use the term to refer to the many localized groups that addressed potential radiation contamination of school lunches.

Mobilizations to demand safe school lunches might seem to be a good way to rally many citizens and to offer an entry point for a broader antinuclear movement. The issue is about children, and about a rare instance in which eating is compulsory (Japanese school lunches are in principle mandatory and students have to eat them, as I discuss in more detail below). However, the safe school lunch movement, which was highly feminized, encountered strong criticism for *fūhyōhigai* (harmful rumors).

How did the women in the safe school lunch movement try to respond to the criticism of fūhyōhigai? This chapter considers strategies of social mobilization in the context of food policing. I point out three salient frames that these women used in framing their activism. First, they turned to science, demanding more scientific data and technical sophistication. Second, continuing a long history of maternalism in women's collective mobilizations, women in the safe school lunch movement emphasized their position as mothers, framing the school lunch safety issue as maternal as well as scientific. The third framing did not emphasize the idea of women as mothers as much as it drew on the increasingly popular discourse of "*joshi* power," which portrayed women as empowered and resourceful, yet appropriately feminine citizen-subjects. (The term "joshi" literally means "women" in Japanese; I explain its more specific usage below.)

How did these women's appeals to science, motherhood, and joshi power influence the politicization of the movement? The safe school lunch movement's criticism of the nuclear village (*genshiryokumura*)—the powerful alliance of the utility industry, the government, and scientists— was relatively muted. It can be contrasted with a more politicized women's movement that emerged after the accident, which took direct actions against the nuclear village (Slater 2014). For instance, the Association of Women for Postnuclear was established in the fall of 2011, and the group has been much more vocal about the need to phase out nuclear power and the accountability of TEPCO and government regulatory bodies. These activists target the core of the nuclear village by organizing sit-ins and rallies, including the Hundred Women's Sit-In by Antinuclear Women of Fukushima and the Sit-In by Women Nationwide in front of the Ministry of Economics and Trade, which has promoted nuclear power in coalition with other powerful actors in the country (Onuma 2012). Surprisingly, many groups in the safe school lunch movement did not build strong relationships with such groups. Furthermore, in contrast to the antinuclear groups' demands, the safe school lunch movement largely remained focused on technical issues, particularly the need for measurement programs.

Safe school lunch movements were situated in a challenging political context in which conservative groups were increasingly powerful, which some analysts called "the right-wing turn" (Nakano 2014) of Japan in the 2000s. At the time of the accident, Japan was under the Democratic Party, which had briefly captured power from the long-ruling Liberal Democratic Party, but the LDP quickly took charge again, voted in by a large margin in the 2012 election. The media were also increasingly conservative, with heightened visibility of the so-called *netto uyoku* (Internet-based right wing) and some mainstream media outlets such as the newspaper *Yomiuri Shinbun*—whose owner was instrumental in founding the postwar Japanese nuclear industry (Nakano 2014). These media accelerated their criticism of antinuclear messages and citizen mobilizations around the nuclear accident.

Schools were a particular object of vigilance by conservative groups as a moral battleground as schools and parents of school-aged children were also seen as the foundation for the fight against the decay of the traditional family. For instance, antifeminist groups mobilized around what they construed as extremist sex education driven by the feminist agenda since the mid-1990s. Furthermore, as Wakakuwa and Fujimura-Fanselow (2011, 342) observed, contemporary mothers were often marked as the source of a societal problem as they were excessively "nagging" and "interfering." It is not hard to imagine the ways in which these social dynamics made it extremely difficult for mothers to raise their radiation concerns with school authorities.

Science and technology studies and feminist literatures have pointed out that turning to science and femininity for social mobilization in technical-scientific controversies can have both enabling and disabling effects. On the one hand, there are cases of successful women's mobilization using citizen science and popular epidemiology. For instance, women in Love Canal near Buffalo, New York, were successful in getting public recognition of contamination and holding the corporations accountable (Newman 2001; Gibbs and Levine 1982; Blum 2008). On the other hand, as summarized in the introduction, theorists of citizen science have shown that it is not necessarily linked to larger social movements, and might instead serve neoliberal interests. Feminist theorists have also noted that the strategic use of femininity can backfire, as it can reinforce gender stereotypes and limit the scope of issues that women can legitimately raise. By analyzing the safe school lunch movement, this chapter extends the analysis of the role of gender in complicating the possibility of citizen science in contamination issues.

School Lunch Programs and Their Vulnerability to Contamination

American readers might think that an easy solution to the threat of contaminated school lunches is available, as children should be able to bring lunch from home or avoid the high-risk items on the menu. But the Japanese school lunch program differs from its US counterpart in that it is considered part of the curriculum and hence participation in it is mandatory for all students.

The postwar school lunch program in Japan started as one of the government antipoverty and malnutrition programs that grew out of post–World War II food aid from the United States under the Licensed Agencies for Relief in Asia and Government Appropriation for Relief in Occupied Areas program. Similar to the American school lunch program, which has played an important role in absorbing surplus commodities, US food aid to Japan was tied to the United States' need to increase agricultural exports, and therefore played a geopolitical role as well in the context of the Cold War (Levine 2010; Satō 2005). With Japanese economic development, the school lunch program's mandate shifted over time from antihunger to education. A particularly strong emphasis on food education (*shokuiku*), which takes food as a medium of education, emerged in the 2000s (Kimura 2011). In 2005, the government established the Food Education Law, firmly positioning school lunches as part of shokuiku and the educational curriculum. According to this law, the objectives of the school lunch program are to "teach the contributions of various people to the production of food, to deepen understanding of traditional food, and to foster the spirit of cooperation, in addition to the intake of appropriate nutrition" (Cabinet Office 2008). This shokuiku policy strengthened the role of the school lunch program within the educational curriculum. For instance, the government started a program for school dietetics teachers who would design school lunch menus and conduct shokuiku education.

Class-based stratification also colored the school lunch dilemma. Families who could afford private schools, which were less likely to have school lunch programs, or to move away from the affected areas to avoid possible contamination had fewer concerns with the safety issues of school lunches. Particularly at the elementary and middle school levels, only small percentages of schools are private, accounting for 1 percent of elementary and 7 percent of middle schools in 2011 (Japan Private Schools Education Institute 2014). The large majority of children go to public schools.

In this situation, what did parents and students do? Some parents asked for special permission for their children to bring homemade lunches or to refuse food items that they deemed risky. The Japanese school lunch program usually serves milk daily, and because of the experience of the Chernobyl accident, many parents did not want their children to drink milk. There are no comprehensive statistics on the prevalence of such solutions, but newspaper reports show that some, but not many, students were able to get permission from the school authorities to opt out of all or part of the school lunch program. In Iwaki City in Fukushima, for instance, 1,800 elementary and middle school children (out of about 30,000 students) did not drink milk in 2012 (interview with the Division of School Lunch and Food Education, Iwaki City, 2014). Some parents also asked the schools to exempt their children from school lunches altogether and allow them to bring homemade lunches. For instance, a survey by the Fukushima City Education Council in February 2013 found, in addition to 204 elementary and middle school students who did not drink milk, 49 students who brought their own rice, and 4 who did not eat school lunches at all ("Gyūnyūnomazu Beihan Wa Jisan" 2013).

Most of the time, the exemptions were allowed on an individual basis without official policy changes. Only some municipal governments granted formal permission.[1] The individual exemption was welcomed by some parents, but many felt that it was not an ideal solution. There was concern about potential teasing or bulling by peers if some children brought bentō lunch and ate something different from the other students. Making homemade lunches every day was also time consuming, making it something only a few parents could afford to do. In addition, individual exemption meant that only the children of concerned parents were protected from contaminated foods.

Parental concerns were also driven by structural factors that seemed to make school lunches more vulnerable to contamination. Neoliberal reform has transformed the school lunch program profoundly since the 1980s, subjecting it to severe cost pressure. In 1985, the Ministry of Education issued a decree on rationalization of the school lunch program, promoting outsourcing to the private sector and the use of consolidated food preparation centers over in-school preparation. The overall fiscal health of local municipalities also deteriorated due to the bursting of the bubble economy, the subsequent decline in tax revenue, the aging population, and increasing social service costs. The Ministry of Home Affairs instructed municipalities to reduce the number of public servants during an administrative reform in 1994, which pressured municipal governments to reduce the number of kitchen staff ("Gōrikatsūchi" 1999). On the other hand, there are families that cannot afford to pay school lunch fees, which are on average 4,100 yen (about US $40) per month (Ministry of Education, Culture, Sports, Science and Technology 2010). According to the Ministry of Education's 2012 survey, about 1 percent of students were not paying the school lunch fee (Ministry of Education, Culture, Sports, Science and Technology 2012).[2] The fiscal difficulties of both local municipalities and parents make school lunches highly cost sensitive.

After the nuclear accident, the price of food from the affected areas declined. Because the school lunch programs had become very cost sensitive, the lower prices made these foods potentially attractive as ingredients for school lunches. Some observers noted that the cesium beef ended up in school lunches precisely for this reason (Kitamura 2011).

Furthermore, the economic stake in the school lunch program is significant, given its size and regularity, and so the program is also subject to industry pressure. Nationwide, 98 percent of public elementary schools and 78 percent of public middle schools provide school lunches—more than 30,000 schools in all (Cabinet Office 2013a).[3] The size of the industry is estimated to be $4.7 billion annually ("Gakkōkyūshoku No Shijōkibo" 2008). Therefore, producers have a huge stake in having their foods served as part of school lunches.

To give an example, one food item that was heavily contaminated by the nuclear accident is mushrooms. Mushrooms were likely to absorb cesium from the logs they grew on, and they were one of the foods that appeared constantly on the government contamination list. Seeing the reputation of their products decline sharply, producers countered by holding a "mushroom day" at Tokyo public schools, conducting classes on the nutritional benefits of mushrooms and donating mushrooms for school lunches that were fed to more than 29,000 kids in 2014. The project was partially funded by the Forestry Agency, which had budgeted $20 million of a government counter-fūhyōhigai program for "mushroom emergency rejuvenation and restoration" ("Genbokuhoshishītake" 2014).[4]

In summary, after the accident, a number of factors seemed to make the school lunch program vulnerable to contamination threats. Its mandatory nature made it a rare case of food that the consumers had no choice but to eat. Its cost sensitivity was worrisome in an environment of declining market prices of food from the affected areas. And because the school lunch program's economic as well as symbolic value was high, industry groups were likely to exert pressure to get their foods incorporated into school lunches. It was in this context that the safe school lunch movement emerged.

Fūhyōhigai Criticisms and the Movement's Focus on Technical Issues

I interviewed the leaders of five groups (two in Tokyo, one in Kanagawa, and two in Fukushima) that were active on school lunch safety issues to ask about their experiences of fighting to get the municipal governments and the school authorities to recognize the risk and take countermeasures. The groups were all founded after the accident. The interviewees were all female, and the groups' memberships were also heavily female, although some fathers took part in them as well.

The first group that I want to discuss was in Kanagawa Prefecture. The experiences of its leader, Katsuma Yoriko, closely resemble the experiences of the other group leaders I talked to in that, despite their nominal successes in making the issue of school lunch safety visible, they have been subject to harsh criticism for fūhyōhigai.

Katsuma-san is a stay-at-home mother, the wife of a "salary man"; their daughter was in elementary school at the time of the accident. Kanagawa Prefecture is located to the south of Tokyo, more than a hundred miles away from the Fukushima nuclear power plants. The government and mass media said that areas like hers, which are miles away from the reactors, were safe, but she was worried. When the new academic year started in April 2011, she expected that the schools would perhaps even cancel the school lunch program.

Surprised that school life went on as if nothing had happened, she called the principal and then the school board to ask that the school lunches avoid food from the affected areas. When I interviewed her in 2014, I asked her how the school authorities responded to her calls. She said she was brushed off as if she were crazy. Undeterred, she started a signature drive to ask the school to measure the contamination level of school lunch foods. She was able to collect close to 2,000 signatures in April and May 2011. She submitted the signatures to the city government, but it rejected the demand, citing the high cost of testing the food.

In July, Katsuma-san heard about the cesium beef scandal. She tried to find out the place of origin for the beef purchased by the school lunch program in her city. When she got the data, some columns were blacked out, which made her highly suspicious. With the help of a local councilman, she tracked the information down, and found out that the city had indeed used the cesium beef in school lunches. She was horrified, and the news shocked many other parents. Her group started a signature drive again, this time collecting more than 7,000 signatures; they submitted their petition to the city legislature in August 2011. The petition asked that the city regularly measure radiation in major food items in school lunches, as well as radiation levels in the air and soil in schoolyards and in school swimming pools. The city had to respond. In October, it started testing ingredients for the school lunch program.[5]

Despite her group's success, Katsuma-san said in the interview that she also experienced fūhyōhigai criticism. The city was following the national government's position that citizens should not be concerned with food safety, even after the cesium beef scandal. For instance, the city newsletter released a special issue on radiation contamination, which cited an expert who said, "Beef contaminated with radioactive cesium over the standard stirred a controversy. However, the standard is not a clear boundary between danger and safety, so you don't have to worry about health impacts even when eating contaminated beef temporarily" (Karaki 2011). The Education Council similarly downplayed the risk of radiation in food, saying, "Even eating [cesium beef] one hundred times would be the same exposure as a single X-ray and there would be no impact on health" (Association to Protect Children from Radiation in Yokohama 2011).

Katsuma-san's group felt profound disapproval from the wider society. First of all, she and her friends felt that they were not taken seriously by the city government. She said in the interview: "They thought I was stupid [bakani sareta kanji]. We were just mothers, not scholars, and they were like, 'it is housewives' hysteria.'" Even her neighbors and many other parents did not want to cooperate with her. She went to talk to the Parent-Teacher Association (PTA) of her daughter's school when she was starting the signature drive, but the parents who held positions in it did not want to upset the school authorities. Originally established by the occupying forces after the war and still under the tight control of the government, PTAs in Japan have historically been conservative, rarely going against the government or school administrative policies (Fujita 1984). The same was true of her neighborhood association, of which she had high expectations; she had thought that the elderly members who held key positions in the association would understand her worry because they would recollect the experiences of the atomic bombs and the Chernobyl accident. But they "totally disliked the idea." It was mainly through the Internet that she was able to connect with other concerned parents in various parts of the same city. Overall, "There was a sense that you could not say what you thought because you would get criticized for fūhyō[higai]," she said.

Katsuma-san's case points to the pervasive influence of the fūhyōhigai discourse and how women who tried to alert the public were chastised in the name of countering harmful rumors. Her group's experience was not unique; it was echoed in the other interviews that I conducted with women in the school lunch movement. For instance, women in another group in Fukushima told me the following story. When they collected signatures to be submitted to the local government, the official petition had to list the real name of one of the members as a representative of the group. Using that name, an anonymous critic posted personal information about the member, including her address and photos of her house, on the web; the member also received anonymous faxes criticizing the group's actions as fūhyōhigai. When the members went to the police because they felt their safety was endangered, the police were not sympathetic at all, telling them, "You must have known that these things would happen, so we should give *you* crime prevention instruction."[6]

These women had to navigate layers of tension. Not only did there exist strong fūhyōhigai sanctions after the nuclear accident, but, specifically in regard to the role of mothers in schools, the last decade has seen a surge in media criticism of what are called *monsutā pearento* (monster parents) or *kurēmā* (claimer) parents. These are parents, often implicitly mothers, who complain excessively and make selfish demands of teachers and school administrators (Honma 2007; Ishikawa 2007; Saito 2010; Yamazaki 2008). The women's wariness about voicing their concerns might also have been increased by the fear that they could easily be categorized as such selfish and overreacting parents.

On a broader level, their experience is a reflection of the larger trend of the fūhyōhigai discourse that I examined in chapter 2. Even when the food in question was so public and something that young children—who are known to be vulnerable to radiation—had to eat, the fūhyōhigai discourse ruthlessly targeted those who raised concerns. Women who voiced their concerns were often portrayed as hysterical and irrational people who did not understand the science of nuclear physics or the principles of radiation protection.

Turning to Science

As anthropologist David Slater and his collaborators noticed in their interviews with young mothers in Fukushima, the nuclear accident imposed a strong social pressure on women to remain silent (Slater, Morioka, and Danzuka 2014). The women in the safe school lunch movement broke the silence at significant cost, and had to find ways to cope with severe fūhyōhigai criticism. Turning to technical/scientific discourses was one strategy in their effort to navigate the social tensions accelerated by the fūhyōhigai discourse.

This was the strategy that the group in Kanagawa relied on. In our interview, Katsuma said that one of the ways that her group tried to counter fūhyōhigai was to frame the issue as a technical and scientific matter. The experience of being brushed off as hysterical housewives made them look for ways to authenticate their voices. They decided that they "would not chant [*shupurehikōru wo ageru wakedemonai*]"; they would "just bring data to explain that this is the reason why we think beef should not be served in school lunches" and "study really hard and try to talk dispassionately." Despite being laypeople without much prior knowledge on nuclear issues, they learned to arm themselves with scientific literature and they tried to talk with government officials and school administrators "dispassionately," drawing on the image of science as a neutral-objective activity and fitting themselves into that image.

My other interviews and reports by others similarly suggest that technical issues were emphasized in the core demands of the safe school lunch movement. Overall, the safe school lunch movement made the institutionalization of testing central to their activism, focusing their work on details such as sampling and frequency. Indeed, one of the challenges faced by the school lunch movement was that, while schools might start testing foods used in the school lunch program, the devil was in the details. For instance, typically, not all foods used were tested due to budget and time constraints, and so the citizen groups had to be vigilant about sampling and frequency. Some municipalities just tested the entire meal as one sample, and some measured contamination levels in several but not all ingredients.[7] They also had to watch the precision of measurement, particularly in terms of the issue of minimum detectable concentration (MDC). The detectors that the national government provided to seventeen prefectures had an MDC of 40 Bq/kg (Makishita 2013, 45), but many groups felt that this MDC was too high (Mothers' Group to Investigate Early Radiation Exposure 2013a). Some groups therefore focused on lowering the MDC used by municipalities. In Kanagawa, for instance, a group mobilized to lower the MDC to 3 Bq/kg (Yoshizawa 2011). Another group in Tokyo learned that their ward was introducing a detector whose MDC was 30 Bq/kg and lobbied to get a better detector with an MDC of 10 Bq/kg ("Onajikondatede Bentō" 2012).

An additional issue that the movement often brought up was the decision to use contaminated food or not after it was measured. In November 2011, the Ministry of Education issued a notice saying that the standard for school lunches should be 40 Bq/kg and if food tested above it, the schools should not use it ("Kyūshokuni Hōshanōkijyun" 2011).[8] The implied message was that if food tested lower than 40 Bq/kg, it could be used in school lunches even if it contained radioactive materials. Indeed, there were cases of municipal governments using food with some contamination but below 40 Bq/kg. For instance, Sendai City in Aomori Prefecture found 11 Bq/kg in a sample of mushrooms and still fed them to the children.[9] Many groups therefore tried to pressure municipal governments to adopt stricter cutoff points.[10]

Some school lunch movement groups also problematized the measurement programs' testing for only limited types of radionuclides. Almost all detectors used by municipal school lunch programs are scintillation detectors that can only detect radionuclides that emit gamma rays such as iodine and cesium, but not others such as strontium that do not emit gamma rays. The government surveys of soil and the ocean have found deposition of strontium due to the nuclear accident, although they argue that strontium has only been found within the range of what was observed during the 1960s when atmospheric nuclear tests were at their height (Ministry of Education, Culture, Sports, Science and Technology 2012).[11] Some groups nevertheless lobbied for the measurement of these noncesium radionuclides, albeit with full awareness of its difficulty and cost.

These technical issues of the structure, precision, and scope of the measurement programs constituted the core agenda of the safe school lunch movement. Given the nature of the contamination, which is invisible and not identifiable by normal human senses, perhaps it is not surprising that the means to make it visible—measurement—became central to the movement's agenda. However, the gendered nature of food policing also needs attention in thinking about the dynamics of this movement and the responses to it. As explained in chapter 2, fūhyōhigai implied a lack of scientific capacity and literacy on the part of the concerned, and women were often blamed for it. The prevailing stereotype of women as weak on technical issues—recall how Katsuma-san talked about being called a hysterical housewife—pressured women to compensate for their perceived lack of competence by turning to science to make the issue visible.

Maternalism in the Safe School Lunch Movement

In January 2014, a group called All Japan Parents Who Want Safe School Lunch organized a meeting with bureaucrats from the ministries of health and economics to push for further policy improvements to en-sure that school lunches were not contaminated due to the nuclear di-saster ("Hōshanōosen No Gakkōkyūshoku Hahaoyatachiwa Genkai Ni Kiteiru" 2014). Speaking to a row of stern-looking bureaucrats in dark business suits, several mothers in plain clothing spoke about their daily struggles to obtain safe food and their concerns about the contamina-tion of school lunches. Irritated by diplomatic official responses that sounded rather rehearsed, one woman pleaded, "Please listen to the voices of mothers. Mothers are the doctors of children," asking them to take se-riously the mothers' wishes for better testing and the avoidance of foods that are likely to be contaminated.[12]

Many other women in the safe school lunch movement often em-phasized their motherhood. When facing fūhyōhigai criticism, women strategically deployed motherhood in their attempts to become legiti-mate speakers on the issue of food contamination. They framed their concerns as reflecting their prioritization of children's health and life. Motherhood can be seen as a crystallization of the opposite of what the fūhyōhigai discourse implies—the concept of a rationally calculating neoliberal subject who prioritizes economic logic—by embodying the logic of life and reproduction, which are perceived as feminine matters.

Several of the groups invoked motherhood as a strategy against fūhyōhigai. One group in Fukushima provides a particularly good exam-ple of the strategy of maternalism. This group was led by a stay-at-home mother, Kakuta Mayumi. After March 11, she asked the school whether her children could bring a homemade bentō lunch instead of eating the school lunch. Luckily, she got permission from the principal. But she feared that bringing bento might invite bullying and stigma for her children in the atmosphere of fūhyōhigai bashing. So she tried to match what was served at school, studying the menus provided by the school. Mimicking the school lunch menu every day was hard; in the interview she said jokingly that she used to hate cooking but the Fukushima accident forced her to be an avid cook, often learning new dishes by necessity. "One item [in the school lunch] that I did not know about was *giseidōfu* [tofu omelet]—I had never cooked it! So I would call the school dietitian and ask her how to make it." Such a private food struggle, however, is lonely and stressful. Seeing that mothers like her were depressed and stressed out because they could not talk about their worries in an environment filled with fūhyōhigai criticism, Kakuta-san started a gathering of mothers at her house, calling it a "smiling mothers' café." Eventually, she expanded to more public mobilizations, starting a signature drive to demand a safety system in the school lunch program by establishing the Mothers' Group to Investigate Early Radiation Exposure.

As explicit in Kakuta-san's choice of the names of her groups, which both use the word "mothers," motherhood was central in this group's framing of their movement. In their interaction with government authorities, they emphasized maternal commitment and the love of children. For instance, in a negotiation with the mayor in February 2013, Kakuta-san astutely observed the machismo in the rhetoric around reconstruction and contrasted it with their maternal identity that prioritized children's safety: "From the government, media, and posters, we often see words like *genki* [cheerful] and *ganbaru* [let's work hard] for the future, but we wonder what substantiates these slogans because we don't feel like there are sufficient means to protect children's safety, and without that, *we mothers* do not feel that this place can be reconstructed."[13] A letter the group addressed to the mayor of their city similarly framed the issue in relation to women's positions as mothers. It said, "mothers who are concerned with the future of children are very worried about radiation exposure by children. . . . Please use food from places where the radioactive materials from the accident did not reach until mothers have evacuated with children to outside the prefecture and until many mothers' worries disappear" (Mothers' Group to Investigate Early Radiation Exposure 2014). It is not that they disingenuously marketed themselves as mothers—even when talking among themselves, they talked about how mothers know best what was going on at school, and so they had to relay their *omoi* (thoughts and feelings) to the authorities.

What about fathers? Many fathers were far from indifferent. But they were constrained by their culturally expected position as the breadwinners and their structural proximity to the economics embedded in the fūhyōhigai discourse. For instance, Kakuta-san talked about seeing that many of her friends' husbands did not support what their wives were doing, or their support often wavered. She wrote on her blog about how difficult it would be for fathers to be on the front lines of this battle in a public space:

> We have to understand that while fathers share the same desire to protect children, fathers face various difficulties in society. Fathers feel the need for reconstruction also to support their families' . . . social position [*shakaiteki tachiba*]. And their position as fathers. We cannot ask fathers to say that protecting children is more important than economic recovery and bear the full brunt of public criticism. . . . Because of their position, it is perhaps to be expected that the vast majority of fathers cannot criticize the problem [of school lunches]. (Mothers' Group to Investigate Early Radiation Exposure 2013b)

Other studies on social dynamics after the Fukushima accident have also shown how men are constrained by hegemonic masculinity to prioritize their roles as breadwinners (Morioka 2014). Such an identity made it difficult for them to problematize radiation risk when the fūhyōhigai discourse portrayed such actions as economically devastating. Therefore, fathers tended to see women's fear of contamination as troublesome, as it hampered economic recovery (Morioka 2014). If patriarchy generally excludes women from public space and limits them largely to domestic space, paradoxically, men's public roles can inhibit them from speaking honestly as concerned fathers. In contrast to the fathers who uphold their social position by not speaking up in society, mothers can be at the forefront.

As Nancy Naples (2014) discussed in the concept of "activist mothering," motherhood is often central to women's activism and can create spaces for women to be active on public issues. Motherhood as an identity is also helpful in authenticating women's voices as driven by maternal love for their children. Like many other social and environmental movements, antinuclear movements have used maternal identity as a strategic position from which to criticize nuclear weapons and nuclear power (Eschle 2013; Managhan 2007).

These gendered constraints and opportunities find ample echoes in previous generations of the antinuclear movement in Japan, when women mobilized as housewives and mothers. In the 1950s, it was a group of housewives in Tokyo who started collecting signatures to protest nuclear tests after the United States dropped a test bomb on Bikini Atoll in the Marshall Islands. The positioning of mothers in this early wave of the antinuclear movement was perhaps clearest in a women's group called the Mother's Congress, which was part of the major Japanese antinuclear organization Gensuikyō. The Mother's Congress motto was, "Mothers who create life want to nurture and protect life."

Maternalism was salient in the later movements of the 1970s–80s, too. For instance, a best-selling book by a housewife, Kansho Taeko, *If It Is Still Not Too Late* (*Mada Maniaunara*) was instrumental in mobilizing previously apolitical housewives in the antinuclear movement (Kansho 1978; Honda 2003; Tajima 1999). In the book, Kansho wrote about the danger of nuclear power, proclaiming that it was fundamentally against the maternal commitment to child and family well-being. Writing as a concerned mother, she lamented, "What a sad age we are living in. Did we ever have a mother who adds poison to everyday meals fed to her child and her family? Poison, even a little, would surely have effects in several years and several decades. Mothers do little about it and can do little about it. We try choosing the least poisonous food. Joyous meal preparation for our families is turned into a burden, making us feeling guilty" (2). Historian Suga Hidemi pointed to a similar maternalism in the 1980s movement by housewives (Suga 2012). One example he cited was Obara Ryoko, a housewife from Ōita Prefecture who came to be called the Joan of Arc of the antinuclear movement. Emphasizing the maternal instinct, Obara wrote, "I had been concerned about large economic development and environmental destruction. In general, many mothers of children are usually concerned about the current situation. We might not speak up, but a concern still exists, forcing us to ask, 'Is this really good? Will the Earth continue to exist?' and 'Is nuclear power really good?'" (cited in Suga 2012, 85). Similarly, in the wave of antinuclear activism that followed the Chernobyl accident, groups often turned to maternal identity to legitimate their cause. For instance, a group called Women's Group to Eliminate Nuclear Power and Bombs was inspired by a project by Finnish women who declared that they refused to have babies unless the government closed all the nuclear power plants in the country. After collecting significant donations within a short span of time, the Japanese group posted advertisements in major newspapers that featured a painting of a mother and child with the heading, "Ash of death is not selective" (*shi no hai wa hito wo erabanai*), surrounded by the names of 5,000 women (Aoyanagi 2012).

Post-Fukushima Japan similarly saw women using their maternal identity to justify raising their voices against the dominant rhetoric of control and safety. Food policing that censored concern about food safety as spreading harmful rumors, hurting producers, and obstructing disaster recovery increased the need for the protective armor that maternal identity could provide. With motherhood positioned as the antithesis of fūhyōhigai discourse with its strong economism and machismo, maternal identity helped women highlight the need for a different kind of logic in thinking about contamination's impacts.

Acting as Joshi

In the September 2013 issue of VERY, a women's fashion magazine, an article on radiation contamination titled "Why I Care about Becquerel-Free Food" ("Bekurerufurī No Kodawari" 2013) appeared amid pages devoted to high-end clothing and makeup tips. The article's visuals were colorful and stylish—all the women in the photos wore fashionable clothes, had their hair nicely done, and looked like they were having a party. But the topic was serious. The women featured were members of a group in Tokyo active on school lunch safety issues. There was also a picture of a detector, and the article mentioned that the women had learned to operate it to measure radiation levels themselves.

The group was started by three mothers, one of whom had called her child's school about the safety of school lunches, to be told simply that the lunches were safe as they did not violate government standards. Infuriated, they started actively lobbying the city government and established the Association to Protect Children in their ward. One of the first major actions they took was to write a letter to the head of their ward in June 2011, asking him to lobby the Ministry of Health and Welfare to make the standards stricter, to request dairy companies to check the radiation concentration level of milk, and to measure the contamination levels in schoolyards. In fall 2011, they started a signature drive to demand a testing system for school lunches, and they successfully collected more than 18,000 signatures. As a result, the ward purchased two detectors and started testing sample meals in April 2012. At the mothers' request, the ward also started posting information on its webpage about where the food used in lunches came from.

When I interviewed one of the leaders, I asked her about the VERY article. She said it was highly strategic. The article's photo of a detector and the mention of the *rike-jo* (scientific women) members who had acquired knowledge and skill in radiation measurement were not accidental. They insisted that the magazine include the photo of the detector in the article. Emphasizing their technical and scientific focus, the group strategically showcased their technical competence.

But the interviewee said that not only the technical emphasis but the choice of VERY itself was strategic. They did not want to be featured in left-leaning newspapers and magazines, but in a regular women's magazine. VERY is focused primarily on fashion (similar to *Vogue* and *Elle* in the United States) and as one of the largest women's fashion magazines in Japan, with a readership of about 260,000, it is quite mainstream. The group wanted to show that activists could be like them—ordinary women—because they wanted to change the stereotypical image of activists as poor, committed to nothing but their activism, exhausted, and worn out by struggle.

The example of the VERY article indicates a different kind of strategy being tried by Japanese women, which I call activist joshi. The term "joshi" would be simply translated as "woman" in English, but it bears a distinct connotation since the late 1990s when it started to be used in the phrase *joshi ryoku*, or "joshi power" (Baba and Ikeda 2012). Like the American concept "girl power," the term conjures women's and girls' power and comradery but also of hipness and consumerism. An activist joshi then can be understood as a woman who becomes socially active but identifies herself as a woman with joshi power in the new millennium. Activist joshi might be mothers, but their emphasis in their self-presentation is more on resourceful femininity than maternal devotion. They are less likely to resort to reproduction as a uniting theme among women and are more inclusive of young women and nonhousewives.

Because of its departure from the traditional mother image, the activist joshi might seem to fully shed the patriarchal constraints on women.

Yet a closer scrutiny reveals that, akin to the US girl power discourse, joshi power celebrates the power of women and their camaraderie, but the image of these empowered girls or women still resides squarely within hegemonic standards of beauty and acceptability. The prevailing joshi discourse tends to fall short of feminist politics in still implicitly affirming traditional gender stereotypes and norms that emphasize beauty and traditional femininity.[14]

In order to consider the implications of the emergence of activist joshi as a new strategy for activist women, it needs to be situated against the backdrop of the postfeminist gender settlement (McRobbie 2009). As explained in the introduction, the postfeminist gender settlement refers to the idea that a pretense of gender equality (that is, postfeminism) paradoxically exacerbates the gendered demands on women to be resourceful yet nonthreatening. Importantly, the settlement nullifies the need for women to collectively mobilize, as the assumption is that structures of injustice no longer exist. Perhaps the most prominent example of the domestication of women's activism under the postfeminist gender settlement is the pink ribbon campaign for breast cancer, where women's advocacy is reduced to shopping, and the maintenance of hegemonic femininity becomes a symbol of triumphant survivorship, obfuscating possible environmental and industrial causes of breast cancer (Ehrenreich 2001; King 2006; Klawiter 2008). Activist joshi are like those pink ribbon campaigners whose identity resides within the confines of hegemonic femininity, which leads to the taming of their activism because they need to be feminine—always friendly and certainly unthreatening.

Although the group that was featured in VERY does not necessarily count as a case of demobilization of political advocacy, in other cases, embracing the activist joshi discourse evidently has tamed women's activism. Take the example of a project called Peach Heart created by young women from Fukushima. The group's main objective was to help rehabilitate Fukushima. But their activities were framed around hegemonic femininity and focused on beauty and shopping. For instance, they held workshops with the objective of helping women in Fukushima, but their topics have not been the impacts of radiation or getting compensation from TEPCO, as one might imagine, but how to put on makeup and find good boyfriends. The ways in which they have tried to address health threats from the disaster have been similarly framed by hegemonic femininity. When people were wearing masks to reduce their inhalation of radioactive particles, Peach Heart suggested designing "cute" masks that use girlish fabrics instead of plain white. Moreover, while the group has participated in antinuclear conferences, its criticism of the nuclear establishment is diluted by its appearance in one of the utility companies' public relations campaigns.[15] Peach Heart and a related group called the Research Institute of Joshi Life (Joshi no Kurashi Kenkyujo) also exemplify a simultaneous shift toward consumerism as a means of social change. They sold goods such as earrings and other crafts with cute themes, ostensibly to support Fukushima's reconstruction. As in the case of the pink ribbon campaign in the United States, shopping and grooming seem to be the preferred mode of advocacy for activist joshi.[16]

In their analysis of postaccident Fukushima social tensions, David Slater and his collaborators astutely observed that women were ascribed a "politically correct emotion" of fear, but not anger (Slater, Morioka, and Danzuka 2014, 488). This mirrors the requirements of the postfeminist gender settlement, which shuns anger as a distasteful trait of feminism (and of so-called angry feminists) and promotes cheerfulness and friendliness as appropriate emotions for women. Being activist joshi is perhaps one way to perform such cheerful, friendly, and unthreatening femininity while engaging with social issues. But the drawback is that adherence to respectability and hegemonic femininity often muddles political positioning. The confines of hegemonic femininity seem to compel activist joshi to make only a subdued criticism of the nuclear village.[17]

In summary, using the discourses of science, motherhood, and joshi power have been useful strategies for many women in the context of fūhyōhigai and the stringent parameters of acceptability for women under the postfeminist gender settlement. Framing their concerns around science, maternal devotion, and joshi helped ordinary women authenticate their voices in order to get some concessions from the authorities. Yet these strategies all seem to be a double-edged sword. As anthropologist Amy Borovoy said of motherhood in Japan, science, motherhood, and joshi are perhaps the "only role that offers them [women] support, stability, and some measure of social recognition" (2005, 168). Depicting themselves in certain ways may seem necessary to these women to count as good citizens and not be labeled as exhausted and dangerous activists. However, more structural and radical demands might have been muted under the weight of these specific framings of the women's relationships to society. The salience of science, motherhood, and joshi power therefore reflects the still-profound struggles that women face to find public voices on socially controversial issues.

The Case of Local Rice from Fukushima

The safe school lunch movement has achieved some practical policy outcomes that are not insignificant. In some municipalities, groups have been successful in getting the authorities to start to measure contamination levels in school lunches.[18] The national government has also acted. In November 2011, it decided to subsidize the cost of detectors to be used in the school lunch programs in seventeen prefectures.[19] The Ministry of Education also started a school lunch monitoring program in 2012 to track the trend of contamination over time (Makishita 2013, 46).[20]

A curious feature of these achievements, however, was that in most of these cases the government decisions were made without transparent public debates or consultation. Even where school lunch safety groups were already active, they were rarely invited to help formulate the policies. Rather, the government decisions have typically been presented as benevolent concessions by the authorities. As Jacques Rancière (1998) said, policing renders people's voices mere noise; the safe school lunch movement might create enough noise to pressure the government to act, but rarely has been a voice to be acknowledged.

These troubling dynamics became salient with one of the most controversial issues in school lunches after the accident: the use of local rice in Fukushima's school lunch program. In 2013, several cities in Fukushima Prefecture announced that they would use Fukushima rice in school lunches. This was in line with the food education (shokuiku) campaign. Article 3 of the Food Education Law established in 2005 called upon the government and local municipalities to promote, among other things, the use of local food in school lunches. The government revised the School Lunch Law to align it with the Food Education Law by including the promotion of *chisan-chishō* (locally produced, locally consumed) as a function of school lunch programs. In the second Food Education Plan, announced in 2006, the government set the goal of 30 percent local food use in school lunches by 2010. In addition, Fukushima Prefecture was suffering from the decline in sales of its agricultural produce due to the nuclear accident. As a way to support its farmers, the prefecture wanted to resume using local rice in school lunches, and so decided to provide incentives to municipalities. This became a huge controversy.

From the perspective of the farmers and the government authorities, this local rice policy was a sound decision. They like to emphasize that Fukushima rice is actually the safest in the nation. Thanks to a newly developed detector that can scan bags of rice on a conveyer belt at relatively high speed, all rice produced in the prefecture, not only samples, is tested at least once. This is not done anywhere else in the nation. In addition to this comprehensive measurement, samples of rice to be used for the school lunch program are tested two more times—the second time at the rice polishing factory and the third time in the school kitchens. National data also show that detected cases of rice contamination are rapidly declining. In 2013, only twenty-eight cases exceeded the government standard of 100 Bq/kg, out of 1.1 million tests.

But opposition emerged. One mother in Fukushima that I interviewed said, "I wonder if the measurement is sufficient. For us, 'Sorry, that rice had radiation' would be too late. . . . Children were exposed to radiation and the concern about the health impacts will continue for a long time. What I really want is 0 Bq/kg. That is the responsibility of adults." From her perspective, it would be better to take a more cautious approach because the school lunches are eaten by children, and children in Fukushima are generally exposed to relatively high external radiation in their daily lives. Furthermore, while the assumption of safety depends upon the view that the radioactive materials deposited in 2011 are under control and their movements in the ecosystem are predictable, new depositions of radioactive materials are still possible. Indeed, in summer 2014, it was reported that decontamination work at the troubled reactors had caused an additional release of radioactive materials into the atmosphere, resulting in contamination of rice in some areas of Fukushima. Even scientists and agronomists working in Fukushima were caught off guard by this incident because it showed that current farm decontamination and prevention strategies are insufficient if this kind of additional release continues to take place. Another issue is the exclusive focus on cesium. The government standard of 100 Bq/kg factors in the possible existence of noncesium nucleoids such as plutonium and strontium by assuming that they exist at certain percentages relative to cesium. Yet concerned women pointed out that researchers did not have a good understanding of the distribution and movement of plutonium and strontium in the environment and that theoretical values might not reflect reality.

How people evaluate the local rice use policy depended, therefore, upon complicated assessments of radiation threats to human health, the extent of actual contamination, and the possibility of new contamination. Decoding these uncertainties and deciding whether the local rice policy was a good policy is not my focus here. Rather, my point is that more attention should be paid to the process, in addition to the outcome, of policy decision making. The local rice use policy came as a surprise for students and parents. The newspaper reports attributed the policy to strong lobbying by Fukushima farmer groups who suffered from the significant decline in sales of their produce. From the perspective of farmers, the significance of having their rice used in school lunches went beyond the economic benefits—its symbolic value in restoring the image of Fukushima rice was paramount. Asked why they wanted to focus on rice in school lunches, the cooperative's director was quoted in the national newspaper as saying, "When I make a sales pitch [for Fukushima rice], what hurts most is when they say, 'But they don't use it in school lunches'" (Sekine 2013). The school lunch program became a symbolic battleground for the farmer cooperatives to prove the safety of their produce.

The farmers' voices were heard by the authorities, while, in contrast, the women's voices were rendered simply noise. The decision was not made until 2013, well after the groups in Fukushima became active on school lunch safety issues. The government officials and school authorities were well aware of the groups' presence. Yet they proceeded without including these groups, which were then forced to react to the decision post facto.[21]

Science and technology studies scholars have observed that when scientific resolution of a controversy is impractical or impossible, social resolution ought to be sought (Kleinman 2000; Rowe and Flewer 2005; Sclove 2000; Wynne 1992). Yet the local rice policy moved in the opposite direction; the decision was made behind closed doors, no parents were consulted, and explanation came after the fact. It might be suggested that given the nature of Japanese bureaucracy, which is not necessarily famous for transparency, this manner of proceeding was inevitable. But why was it that one party to the debate—farmer cooperatives—was able to be heard by the government, while the activists were not?

The school lunch program deserved a much more comprehensive public debate than it received, particularly because the economic and symbolic stake for the producer groups was evident. In the end, the social legitimacy of the school lunch program suffered because the policy makers failed to include interested parties other than the producer groups in the decision making process.

That so many of the people who were active on the school lunch issue before the decision was made are women should lead us to ask about the gendered dynamics of the situation. The case of the local rice use policy needs to be understood in light of the long history of gendered access to the public sphere. As many feminist scholars have pointed out, access to the public sphere is stratified by social power, and women have historically been excluded from it. If the idealized image of democracy presupposes a public sphere where citizens engage in reasoned deliberation of topics of social importance, the reality of the public sphere is exclusionary to minority groups and women (Fraser 1997).

Education of children is an area where women—particularly mothers—seem to have a uniquely large say in the public sphere. Mothers have been seen as an integral part of education in Japan; during the postwar economic boom, mothers were expected to devote themselves to preparing their children to excel in the competitive *gakureki shakai* (academic pedigree society) and to contribute to the national economy (Allison 1996). Given that more women are educated (12 percent of females went to four-year universities in 1980, 47 percent in 2014) and in the workforce (24 percent of women in the mid-1980s versus 38 percent in 2005–9 continued to work after childbearing) today (Gender Equality Bureau 2015), we might expect that contemporary mothers would be more vocal and empowered to participate in the governance of schools. Nonetheless, neoliberal and postfeminist ideas of a proper citizen-subject exert a strong influence. Mothers who have more education and independence might feel empowered to place individual demands on schools and teachers but be constrained from working collectively to enact change in the shared governance of schools.

In the post-Fukushima landscape, it seems that women were visible but were not considered to be contributing actors in policy decisions.

The abrupt local rice policy decision meant not only that the government was not transparent—it also meant that the government refused to acknowledge women as a legitimate part of the public to be engaged in deciding an important issue.

Conclusion

Countering food policing is a challenge for those on the margins of society, particularly when contaminants are byproducts of a powerful industry. The problem is even more pronounced when the contaminants are invisible and thus depend upon scientific means to be made visible and perceptible. Olga Kuchinskaya's analysis of the Chernobyl nuclear accident took invisibility as the central factor in describing the postaccident situation in Belarus. She found that the invisibility of radiation was maintained and reinforced by government authorities and affiliated experts. Many local people were also constrained from actively undermining the official narrative (Kuchinskaya 2014).

In contrast, the women in the safe school lunch movement in Japan worked to make the issue socially visible, and in some cases they were successful. They voiced their concerns despite the official assurances of safety and they demanded precautionary measures despite food policing. Using different discourses of science, motherhood, and joshi power, they tried to present themselves as reasonable and agreeable citizen-subjects in order to legitimate their role in making the radiation threat visible and in pressing for policy changes.

However, the paradox in the Fukushima accident was that while the issue might be made visible, the women themselves remained invisible as part of the public, the citizenry that had a legitimate stake in societal debate on the issue. The case of the local rice use policy in Fukushima attests to how, even after they became active and mobilized, they were not invited to the table.

Feminist scholars have long observed that women have historically been excluded from public deliberation (Young 2000). Ironically, women are likely to help make an issue public—to "publicize" technoscientific issues (Marres 2007, 721)—and make them perceptible, but they face challenges to becoming the public in democracy. To build upon Kuchinskaya's important work in Chernobyl that highlighted the role of invisibility, I would argue that visibility is not sufficient to counter food policing. Food policing's insidious effect is not only that it creates pressure that makes contaminants socially invisible or a nonissue, but also that it renders certain people's concerns as mere noise, not voices. A prevailing assumption is that controversies create a concerned public that then can participate as stakeholders; but when a controversy creates a group of concerned women, they might be seen as irrelevant or dangerous, and hence not worthy to be stakeholders.

The dynamic is similar to what scholars have observed in democratization movements in which women were crucial in the initial stages of breaking the silence, but marginalized in the subsequent postauthoritarian regimes that they helped to create (Jaquette and Wolchik 1998). This "dislocation of women" (Hawkesworth 2001) is a complex phenomenon, but some scholars have suggested that it is partly due to interest-group-style politics where political parties and lobbying groups proliferate, rather than grassroots groups. If political representation is limited to formally organized, single-issue or single-ideology groups, it tends to marginalize women's grassroots groups. On the other hand, professionalization or "NGO-ization" of women's organizations has had mixed outcomes (Alvarez 2009), with particularly troubling tendencies toward co-optation and domestication (Lang 2001).

The need for societal discussion and dialogue about contaminants is paramount when scientific conclusions cannot be conclusively drawn, as in the case of radiation. But the experience of the safe school lunch movement indicates that the structure of the policy arena is highly significant in whether decision making includes meaningful dialogue and different voices. Because food contamination issues tend to involve scientific contention and economic consequences, they also tend to have two vocal groups of stakeholders: scientific/industry experts and food producers. But if deliberation is limited to these highly organized groups, it shuts out those who are not able to organize to the same extent. Yet whether decision-making processes make a space for less organized groups—like the women in the safe school lunch movement—ultimately shapes the social legitimacy of the outcome of the deliberation.

FOUR

Citizen Radiation-Measuring Organizations

Measuring Station in the Forest is the name of a citizen radiation-measuring organization (CRMO) to the northwest of Tokyo. It is one of the many CRMOs that emerged in Japan after the Fukushima nuclear accident, where citizens can bring their own food to be tested for cesium concentrations. Its leader is Tsuchida Kanako, a housewife in her sixties. Tsuchida-san, along with several other women who, as mothers and grandmothers, became concerned about radiation's impacts on children, bought a detector, learned how to operate it, and established the CRMO as a nonprofit organization in 2013. Many people bring food to the CRMO to be tested. By the end of 2013, the CRMO had measured close to 800 samples of food and beverages brought in by citizens in their neighborhood.

Located in a small wooden house that used to be a restaurant, the CRMO was quite spacious and felt comfortable, equipped with a room for children to play in, and another larger tatami room where people could sit and chat, besides the space allotted for the detector. As I walked into the CRMO, I saw for sale, arranged on a wooden countertop, tea, beans, and honey that had been tested for radioactive contamination. I also saw flyers and posters advertising a variety of events—from the screening of a documentary film on Timor Leste's struggle for independence to lectures on radiation risk and antinuclear movements.

The political flyers suggested an antinuclear stance and a connection to broader progressive grassroots movements, so I was particularly struck when, in the interview I conducted with the women at the CRMO, they talked about their fear of being labeled professional activists and emphasized that they did not seek to establish relationships with any political organizations or social movement organizations. As a way to highlight the importance of being seen as nonpolitical, they talked about the time they organized a lecture by a physicist who is famous for his antinuclear stance. A local labor union became involved, which presented a conundrum, as the union could mobilize people quickly, but the women were also wary of being seen as union sympathizers. They eventually decided to work with the union, but with much hesitation. Tsuchida-san, the leader, phrased their fear of stigmatization as the worry that they "would be seen as people who are on that side" (*acchigawa no hito*) if they collaborated with unions. She went on to say, "We did not want to be activists [*katsudōka*]. There is a woman here who has been issuing newsletters on social problems. People see her as strange. She is a professional activist and not a regular person. We need to look for a new way of social movement. We don't want to be called professional activists [*undō no puro*]. We are regular mothers."

Measuring Station in the Forest is not unique. I discovered throughout my interviews with many other CRMOs that they too shunned politics and concentrated on science. This seems counterintuitive. Many observers heralded CRMOs as part of a new wave of activism in Japan, an instance of progressive citizen science and rejuvenated social action after the triple disasters in 2011. But their political orientations are actually far from clear-cut. In the interviews that I conducted, many CRMOs expressed the desire to refrain from "politics" or anything politicized and instead to focus on "science" and "testing."

The conventional view of citizen science assumes, rather than problematizes, its link to politics and social movements. In many cases of citizen science, social movement activists tend to be the ones who collect data and engage with scientists: HIV/AIDS patient activists have worked with medical scientists to change the way clinical trials are done (Epstein 1998); residents have collected water samples in order to push the government to clean up chemical contamination of the land (Brown 1992). In these cases, citizen science is a tool for social movements to achieve their social change goals, and their political motivations are clear. Yet the political involvement of CRMOs in Japan is more complicated than the social movement model might suggest. Obviously, some CRMOs are clearly antinuclear and do not hesitate to be vocal in criticizing the government and TEPCO. But many do not want to engage in explicitly political activism.

This is perhaps something to be expected from Japanese civil society organizations, which scholars have described as docile and nonconfrontational (Pharr 2003). The literature that critically examines citizen science, however, suggests that the CRMO experience might not be totally unique to Japan. Scholars have noted the influence of neoliberalism on social movements broadly, and on citizen science more specifically.[1] Citizen science, in fact, can be a way of outsourcing regulatory functions to the private sector (Jalbert, Kinchy, and Perry 2013). Many scholars are increasingly noting the "nonactivism" (Boudia and Jas 2014) of participants in popular epidemiology and citizen science. The concepts of citizen science and popular epidemiology started with the theorization of social movements that were active for extended periods of time, and that succeeding in gathering data and ultimately having larger structural impacts—therefore, their maturation into full-fledged and sustained mobilization was often taken for granted. But more recent literature shows that their longevity and tenacity is not guaranteed. For instance, in China, geographer Anna Lora-Wainwright (2013) found that villagers did not collectively mobilize to reduce industrial pollution from factories in their villages even after they started gathering scientific information and epidemiological data that could well be used for such actions. In Argentina, Auyero and Swistun (2009) found that shantytown residents did not rise up in protest, even though they had brought in scientists who collected data that indicated air, water, and soil contamination and their impacts on the health status of the residents. In Italy, Laura Centemeri (2014) found that when a chemical factory explosion in Seveso, Italy, exposed residents to carcinogenic dioxin, despite the presence of nonprofit organizations that came to work with them, the local residents did not engage in collective mobilization to seek more information disclosure or prevention. This literature points to important questions to be asked regarding the degree to which citizen science results in radical politics.

This chapter examines the CRMOs and provides a basic profile of seventy-four organizations that emerged across Japan after the Fukushima accident. They are grassroots organizations that are open to ordinary citizens who want to have their food's contamination levels measured by detectors. Who are the actors involved, and what are the CRMOs' challenges and contributions? In addition to explaining the CRMOs' structure and contribution to food safety, this chapter focuses on their politics. How do we explain their seemingly apolitical stance? If many of them do not want to be seen as political and do not want to play an explicit role in the antinuclear movement, what could be their political—in addition to their scientific—contributions?

I argue in this chapter that their professed nonpolitical stance is rooted in an increasingly powerful understanding of the citizen under neoliberalism. Scholars have discussed how calculations of the neoliberal states mutate the notion of a citizen to mean a specific type of citizen-subject (Ong 2003). The care that Tsuchida-san took to differentiate "regular mothers" like herself from "professional activists" reflects a broader pressure on citizens to conform to a particular norm of what a citizen should look like, which is apolitical, docile, and aligned with the neoliberal ideology of productivity and self-responsibility. In this context, citizen science becomes an ideal tool to perform such citizenhood, not only because of the prevailing image of science as neutral and objective, but also because citizen science can be seen as citizens taking care of themselves by using scientific means, which is in line with the neoliberal promotion of self-care. Conversely, marked as the opposite—unproductive, disruptive, or unconstructive—traditional politics is increasingly seen as an inappropriate field for citizens. Such a neoliberal understanding pressures citizen scientists to shift from being activists to being technicians who use science as a means of self-care.

But at the same time, it is important to ask whether citizen science under neoliberalism necessarily always leads to such an apolitical outlook. Are the people who started CRMOs completely domesticated conformists who are content to simply run the detectors? Many indeed concentrate on doing good measurement. But the passion and commitment they bring to the act of measuring suggest that the CRMOs require a careful analysis, rather than simply being dismissed as a refuge from politics; perhaps it is necessary to consider the possibility of a different kind of politics. The case of CRMOs examined here calls for a nuanced understanding of citizen science in the neoliberal era, both as a way to avoid and as a way of doing politics.

CRMOs: Profiles

Citizen radiation-measuring organizations started to emerge several months after the nuclear accident, in the summer of 2011. Earlier, in the 1980s, the Chernobyl accident had inspired the establishment of similar organizations. After Chernobyl, Japan's Ministry of Health and Welfare set a standard for imported food (at 370 Bq/kg of cesium), but they did not make the testing data available, and only disclosed it when the limit was exceeded. This prompted activists to start organizations to monitor food themselves, such as a nonprofit group in Tokyo called the Radiation Contaminated Food-Measuring Room. Similar testing organizations emerged across Japan, but only a few survived longer than a decade (Watanabe 2004). When the Fukushima accident happened in 2011, only a few were still active and continuing to test food. Among them were the Koganei Citizen Measuring Organization and the Radiation Contamination Food-Measuring Room, both in Tokyo. The Koganei Citizen Measuring Organization was a hybrid of sorts, a nonprofit group working with the municipal government. Pressured by concerned citizens, the city government had purchased a detector and paid for its maintenance for more than two decades. The Radiation Contamination Food-Measuring Room was established by the Citizens' Nuclear Information Center, an organization that has been central in the anti–nuclear reactor movement in Japan since the 1970s. A CRMO in Shizuoka called Shizuoka Radiation-Measuring Room was established in 1988.

When the accident took place in March 2011, there were very few places where citizens could bring their own food to be tested for contamination. Most detectors at academic laboratories were not open to citizens. There were some commercial laboratories, but their testing fees were rather expensive. The detector at the Koganei CRMO was not operational as it needed repair. The Citizens' Nuclear Information Center was open to citizens, but it was flooded with requests for tests, particularly from consumer cooperatives. It was in this context that many citizens decided to start their own CRMOs.

The post-Fukushima network of CRMOs started independently of the surviving organizations, although many of their founders paid visits to these forerunners to get tips and practical advice. The first group of post-Fukushima CRMOs was established with help from the French antinuclear group CRIIRAD (Commission de Recherche et d'Information Indépendantes sur la Radioactivité) and coordinated by Kaneda Noboru and Sugita Mariko. Kaneda-san, a musician fluent in English and French, cultivated his international network to gain information and assistance. Sugita-san was a single mother in Tokyo who had been active on peace and health issues. Their initial focus was on contamination of the air, and with the help of CRIIRAD they brought dosimeters to Japan with which they measured air contamination in multiple locations in Fukushima. Realizing that food contamination was a serious concern among citizens, they went to Europe to receive training to measure radiation in food. They came back and helped establish a network of CRMOs, called Citizen Radiation Measuring Stations. Seven CRMOs were established within their network, mostly in Fukushima but also in Tokyo.

Seeing the success of these CRMOs, citizens in other areas started similar ones. As of February 2014, I had identified seventy-four active CRMOs across Japan, from Hokkaido to Okinawa, not only in the areas surrounding the troubled reactors.[2] My assistants and I interviewed members of sixty-five of them.

Many CRMOs were established by lay citizens who had no previous experience in radiation measurement. Most CRMOs use a type of detector called a scintillation detector, or scintillator. A scintillation detector works by sensing when radiation interacts with a material in the detector. Learning to operate this type of detector seemed manageable to the lay citizens who started CRMOs, despite their lack of prior training. The detector usually comes with software that automatically prints out a result, with an estimate of the concentration of radioactive cesium. People at CRMOs learned how to operate the detectors and interpret results by going to workshops offered by nonprofit organizations, or from books, websites, and consultation with the detector manufacturers and other CRMOs. There were some university-affiliated researchers who gave advice to CRMOs as well.

The central objective of CRMOs is to measure the concentration of radioactive materials in food brought to them by citizens. In an effort to gauge this aspect of their contribution, in the interviews I asked how many samples of food they had tested by the end of 2013, and in how many cases they were able to detect contamination. Not all the CRMOs tallied the number of measurements they did, but the total number of food and beverage samples tested by forty-nine CRMOs was more than 60,000. Interviews indicated that some of these tests resulted in the discovery of holes in the government safety system: The CRMOs had found more than a thousand cases of food contaminated by cesium above the government standards (100 Bq/kg).[3]

The CRMOs were particularly instrumental in measuring foods that are not usually measured by the government. For instance, foods produced

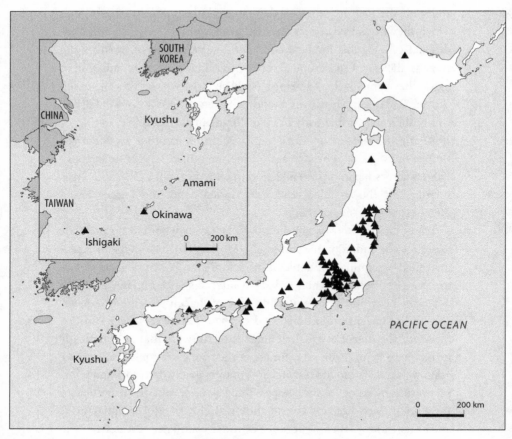

Map 4.1 Locations of CRMOs as of February 2014.

in home gardens and backyards are often consumed by families or exchanged as seasonal gifts, and regular government inspection does not cover them. Wild game, fish, herbs, bamboo shoots, and mushrooms that people hunt, fish, and forage for also tended to fall outside the government measurement schemes. These foods could be brought to CRMOs and checked for contamination.

It would be easy to point to shortcomings of the CRMOs, such as the lack of certified staff members to operate detectors and the uncertainty of ensuring the best conditions for testing. The limitations of the type of detectors they use are also an issue. Due to the higher cost of germanium semiconductor detectors, most CRMOs have scintillators. The former cost about fifteen million yen each, while the latter can cost as little as one million yen. But a scintillator's precision is lower, particularly in measuring concentrations in urine and breast milk (Inoue 2012).

However, while the narrative that takes the shortcomings of CRMOs as definitive is one that privileges the expert point of view, it is also possible to point out that the CRMOs, despite their imperfections, have been able to make important contributions to food governance. There was an undeniable demand from citizens to have better data on the extent of contamination, and CRMOs met this demand by working to fill the post-Fukushima knowledge gap. Not only did they identify hidden cases of contamination that violated government standards, they provided data on lower-level contamination, which many citizens felt was necessary to protect their health.

Types of CRMOs

Who were the people who established these CRMOs? What about their prior experience with social activism? Although the literature on citizen science is full of instances in which social movement activists engage in citizen science, my interviews with CRMOs indicated diverse backgrounds of those involved in them, many of whom had little to no activist experience.

There are at least five patterns that I have identified in regard to the background of core people in the CRMOs. The first group is CRMOs that were started by antinuclear activists who had been active before the Fukushima nuclear accident. One example is the Radiation Monitoring Center for Citizens, in Chikurinsha, in the Kantō region. It was established by a coalition of several antinuclear organizations such as the Association to Think about Aging Nuclear Reactors in Fukushima (Fukushima Rōkyugenpatsu wo Kangaerukai). This association was established in 1995 and has been active in the antinuclear movement, protesting against utility companies about safety issues. Using their preexisting networks, the longtime activists obtained detectors from a US antinuclear group, the Nuclear Information and Resource Service, based in Maryland. The French antinuclear group ACRO (Association pour le Contrôle de la Radioactivité de l'Ouest) also helped this CRMO by sending a technical expert in radiation detection. The international network of antinuclear activism motivated and helped this existing domestic organization to establish a CRMO.

Another CRMO in the Chūbu region also centered on longtime nuclear activists. Among the first of the post-Fukushima CRMOs, it opened its doors in August 2011. Its leader is a female chemist in her sixties who had worked for a prefectural environmental research institute. Part of her job had been to measure radioactive materials resulting from atmospheric nuclear testing, and so she had relevant technical expertise. Even before the Fukushima nuclear accident, she was involved in various antinuclear movements, particularly those opposing nuclear reactors in the Chūbu region, although the organization that she was involved in stopped being active in the early 2000s. When the nuclear accident happened, she got together with her friends from her previous activism and started planning to open a CRMO. They got seed money from an antinuclear group, the Takagi Fund, and asked for more donations from small donors, with which they purchased the detector. Part of the reason why they were able to start early was that their leader knew whom to contact to get hold of a detector, as they were in short supply after the accident.

Although this CRMO was started by seasoned antinuclear activists, most of its twenty or so volunteers did not have much experience with social movements, let alone radiation measurement. I met four staff members. They were all women in their forties to sixties. They talked about how they had not been involved in any political activism. One of them, Tanaka-san, said, "I used to know someone who opposed nuclear power, but we thought she was a bit strange." But the nuclear accident shook her and, like the other three, she felt "she had to do something." This pattern of experienced antinuclear activists working with a group of people who were novices in both science and activism was repeated in several other cases as well.

Some CRMOs were established by people who might not have been involved in nuclear issues, but were engaged in other struggles such as consumer rights, environmentalism, and peace activism, and found the measurement of radiation to be a new site for their activism. For instance, a CRMO in the Kantō region was established by two women who had been active in consumer movements. Both of them were in the Seikatsu Club, which is an alternative consumer cooperative that also sends housewives to local legislative bodies (LeBlanc 1999). One of them had been elected to a municipal council, and she had been involved not only in consumer rights but also environmental education. They were quick to act in the aftermath of the accident. By April 2011, they had already established the Association to Protect Children from Radiation in their city. They pulled money from their personal savings, bought a detector, connected with a younger generation of mothers, and established the CRMO.

In contrast to those people who had social movement experience prior to establishing CRMOs, many CRMO leaders have no such previous movement experience. Among these, many identify themselves as mothers and fathers, and the protection of children was the main motivation behind their establishment of CRMOs. For instance, a CRMO in Fukushima was established by a group of mothers. They lived in an area that was outside of the mandatory evacuation zone but had relatively high levels of contamination. For one reason or another, they could not relocate to a safer place. Recognizing that their children were being exposed to higher than normal external radiation, these mothers felt that the reduction of internal radiation was one of their few options to reduce the health risks. They began to look for vegetables from outside Fukushima because they felt Fukushima produce had a higher risk of contamination. When they realized that it was difficult to do this at regular supermarkets, they started a *marche* (market), procuring and selling vegetables from outside Fukushima. They also acquired a donated scintillation detector to offer testing services at a cost of about $5 per sample. The organizers had been totally apolitical before the Fukushima nuclear accident. In the interview, the leader (a female in her forties) said, "I did not even know that a petition [*seigan*] was different from requests [*yōbō*] and signatures [*shomei*]. I did not even know that a petition needed a legislator's sponsorship!" But the nuclear accident changed her, and she became engaged in running this organization as well as lobbying local governments on issues such as school lunch safety and the need for air conditioning for schools (as the windows needed to be closed to keep contamination out even in the summer).

Fathers also became involved. One CRMO in western Japan is a one-man operation. The organizer is the father of two children, and he works for a municipal government. Worried about the health of his small son, he started to participate in the meetings of various citizen groups. After purchasing a detector with his personal savings, initially concerned only about his own family, he decided to open it for other worried parents. Given his status as a public servant and also to protect his children from any repercussions, he keeps a low profile, receiving samples by mail and at a friend's shop. Most of his clients are women with small children (many of whom were evacuees from Fukushima and neighboring areas). He placed the detector in a room in his apartment that is dedicated to the detector, locked to keep children out, and has air conditioning running constantly to maintain good conditions for testing. He usually tests one sample per day, turning on the detector before he goes to work. He said that he had been "totally nonpolitical" before the nuclear accident—what he had been passionate about was playing computer games and making his own computers.

Another type of CRMO grew out of support groups for evacuees from the affected areas. In general, evacuees from the affected areas were mothers and children. There is a significant concern among evacuees that while they might have fled the contaminated air, they could still be eating contaminated food. Several CRMOs in the west and south of Japan were established to respond to their concerns. These CRMOs tend to have evacuees as clients who bring in food to test, and some of them have evacuees as staff members. For instance, a CRMO in western Japan was established by an experienced union and antiwar activist in his fifties. He was initially involved in helping evacuees from Fukushima. A comment by an evacuee, "We fled from radiation [by evacuation], but radiation enters food which then is following us," made him realize the need for a place to measure contamination in food. At a meeting in November 2011, one participant brought chicken meat from a local supermarket and tested it, with a result of 29 Bq/kg of cesium. That was the deciding moment—"invisible radiation became visible," showing that even in western Japan, contaminated food was being sold and eaten by citizens. With several evacuees (mothers with children who evacuated due to health concerns and relocated to the west) and help from his prior activist network, he established the CRMO, which started to accept samples from citizens in May 2013 (Morita 2012a).

Several CRMOs were established by religious organizations. A Christian relief network called Tōhoku Help is an ecumenical organization established after the triple disasters in March 2011, which started two CRMOs in the northeastern region, one in Sendai in December 2011 and the other in Iwaki in May 2012. One CRMO in the western region is housed in a small room in a Buddhist temple. The temple's monk had been involved in various peace and antinuclear issues. In particular, he had been active in the Inter-Faith Forum for Review of National Nuclear Policy established in 1993. The forum is ecumenical, involving more than three hundred religious people from various sects within Buddhism, Christianity, and Shintoism. It has organized conferences, participated in antinuclear demonstrations, and issued demands to and negotiated with the government in relation to the expansion of nuclear facilities, nuclear accidents, and the protection of rights of reactor workers. The 2011 disasters strengthened the forum members' belief that, as seen in their declaration in 2012, "it is clear that national policies produce abandoned people [kimin]. We who are grounded in dignity of life cannot overlook this situation, as we have to side with the most marginalized" (Inter-Faith Forum for Review of National Nuclear Policy 2012). This monk used his personal funds as well as several friends' retirement money to purchase the detector, starting the CRMO in June 2013.

Another type of CRMO was established by farmers and people who had been involved in food-related businesses, including organic farmers, natural food store owners, and natural food restaurant owners. These people had prided themselves on providing safe, high-quality food, and the nuclear accident prompted them to think about CRMOs because they wanted to make sure that their products were not contaminated. Furthermore, for organic farmers, such measuring quickly became a business necessity to maintain their relationships with consumers. One example of a farmer-initiated CRMO is in Miyagi Prefecture. The (male) farmer had practiced natural farming, but the nuclear accident forced him to quit farming altogether as he felt there was no point in cultivating contaminated soil. He bought several detectors with his own money and opened a CRMO.

In summary, diverse people became involved in CRMOs. The description above should dispel the notion that their emergence was driven by a single ideological conviction, perhaps as part of the existing antinuclear movement or environmentalism. Rather, CRMOs were established by people with various backgrounds, with varying motivations, and both with and without prior social movement experience and connections to existing organizations.

Politics (or Lack Thereof) of CRMOs

In the interviews I conducted with CRMO members, one of the questions I prepared was about whether the members were involved in citizen activities and whether they were engaged in policy matters. Overall, this question was answered with qualified hesitancy. After conducting more than a dozen interviews, it was increasingly clear that the question was not phrased well and the situation was not so clearcut. The muddled answers from my interviewees suggested that there were different understandings of what counts as citizen activities, policy matters, or politics.

There is no doubt that some CRMOs explicitly participate in antinuclear movements and are solidly embedded in a wider network of antinuclear organizations. They organize antinuclear conferences, support antinuclear candidates in elections, and participate in and coordinate actions opposing the restarting of nuclear reactors and various other energy issues. On the other hand, some CRMOs are run by people who are more interested in the praxis of testing than its political aspects and seem to enjoy the do-it-yourself aspect of radiation measurement. People tweak different aspects of testing to see if they can improve its precision and venture into testing different things such as soil, ashes, and clothes. These people tend to have little political engagement.

The majority of CRMOs have some degree of politicization. Many CRMOs might say that they don't do politics as a group, but individual members do. For instance, a CRMO in southern Japan would not even disclose its test results to nonmembers (which is rare among CRMOs), and its leader said that the CRMO had no political mission. Yet one of their staff had long been involved in lobbying the municipal government about testing school lunches and about the issue of debris from the affected areas. Others who work there, including the leader of the CRMO, are also concerned with the extent of the contamination and are highly critical of government policies such as the level of standards and the frequency of testing. Yet they do not want the CRMO to be seen as involved in politics.

The drawing of boundaries between science and politics would not be surprising in the conduct and norms of scientists (Gieryn 1983). It is usually acknowledged that seeming politicized would be a liability for a scientist. But as a citizen, why not do politics? Of course, CRMOs do not want their test results to be seen as biased or distorted due to their political stance. But there are other reasons why many CRMOs shy away from the political, and they need to be situated in the broader political and historical context in Japan.

From the interviews, it became clear to me that many people associate politics with a rigid hierarchical organization, as in labor unions and political parties. That kind of organizational structure is incongruent with what many CRMOs are comfortable with. In one interview, a CRMO leader said, "A different generation depended on organizations. But today is the age of the social [sōsharu], rather than of organizations [soshiki]. Of course, sometimes that can mean unfortunate losses in elections. It's fine that people protest in front of the National Diet, but I feel that we should aim at social revolution [sōsharu kakumei]." In his view, organizational politics might be good for political revolution, but not for social revolution, and he wanted his CRMO to embody the latter.

Furthermore, the old style of political mobilization was understood to demand strong dedication, to the point of social isolation, and to be rigidly hierarchical; in all these ways, it feels out of sync in contemporary society, and a different style of politics has to be sought. One interviewee clearly saw a CRMO as a conscious choice to seek a different kind of politics. He said, "I was born in the sixties, and was told by my parents that I should not be like the Anpo [student movements in the 1960s] generation ever since I was small. I feel that my way to fight is different and that's why I established this CRMO. I just don't feel comfortable with demonstrations and such."

The avoidance of politics was also accelerated by the renewed stigma of the New Left, which has long haunted antinuclear movements and other social movements in Japan. The New Left groups broke away from the Japan Communist Party in the 1950s and became involved in violent clashes with the authorities over the US-Japan security treaty in the 1960s. After the 1970s, their mobilization power dwindled, yet they were involved in various issues such as opposition to construction of the Tokyo International Airport and to the emperor, and labor rights. They are considered terrorist groups by the government and have also been involved in violent and sometimes deadly infighting as well (Apter and Sawa 1984; Steinhoff 2007).

The nuclear disaster brought new energy to both right and left political factions in Japan. As reported by the government's National Public Security Intelligence Agency, the disasters provided opportunities for extremist groups. An agency report issued in 2012 noted that "extremists tried to recruit workers and students through problematizing the employment issue and through volunteer activities in the affected areas" (Public Security Intelligence Agency 2012, 56).[4]

The involvement of the New Left in the antinuclear movement received particular attention as opposing nuclear power became a key element of its platform after the nuclear accident. For instance, a New Left group called Chūkaku-ha established a network called Subeteno Genpatsu Imasugu Nakusō! Zenkoku Kaigi (Let's Abolish All Nuclear Reactors Right Now, known as NAZEN) in August 2011. In addition to challenging the government's nuclear policies, NAZEN was also involved in directly serving the affected people. They conducted donation drives for victims as well as opening a medical clinic in Fukushima ("Fukushima Kyōdō Shinryōjo Wo Kaisetsu" 2013). Chūkaku-ha is considered a terrorist organization by the Japanese police and is known for violent clashes with the authorities since its founding in the 1960s and sometimes bloody internal conflicts known as *uchi-geba*. It is usually seen as a violent extremist group by ordinary citizens and other citizen activists (Ando 2014).

The more mainstream antinuclear movement saw the New Left's post-Fukushima emphasis on nuclear issues ambivalently.[5] Some were wary of any association with extremists, while others accepted the New Left as a welcome ally. For instance, Yamamoto Taro, who ran on the antinuclear independent platform in the general election of July 2013 and received widespread support from progressive and mainstream antinuclear groups, said that he would not reject the support of NAZEN (Ikeda 2013). The New Left was also reputed to be involved in CRMOs. For instance, a CRMO in northeastern Japan purged one of its key members because she was suspected of being a Chūkaku-ha sympathizer, and declared its nonaffiliation with the radical groups. Some CRMOs are also reputed to be related to another leftist group called Movement for Democratic Socialism (MDS), which has also been marked as an extremist group by the government.[6]

The New Left entanglement with environmental mobilization is not unique to the post-Fukushima situation. Take the example of the Minamata struggle, one of the four major environmental contamination cases in the history of postwar Japan, when residents near the Chisso Chemical Corporation suffered from chemical contamination and fought for compensation and cleanup. The Minamata residents organized themselves and negotiated with the company and the local and national governments. Radical students, as well as socialist and communist groups, came to join the struggle, and residents faced a major challenge in keeping control over the movement (George 2001).

While the Minamata residents were ultimately successful in maintaining independence, others have not been. The movement opposing the construction of the Tokyo International Airport since the 1960s, for instance, was originally centered on farmers who refused to give up their land for the airport, but radical student movements started appearing at the protests and sit-ins. The farmers were initially careful to retain their autonomy but later were overshadowed by the radical movement (Apter and Sawa 1984). Historian Timothy George writes, "Whereas the radical students in Narita proceeded to 'swallow up' the farmers' protest for their own purposes, the Minamata movement, like the consumers' movement, was able to attract more mainstream support" (2001, 281–82).[7]

Given this history, it is not a surprise that some people involved in CRMOs were worried about being similarly hijacked by the radical groups. There were rumors of New Left groups collecting funds and recruiting new members in the name of CRMOs. It is unclear to me how the New Left actually exploited these CRMOs. Some interviewees said that the New Left was involved in CRMOs for the purpose of *orugu* (a transliteration of "organizing," meaning to recruit new members) and channeling the funds collected for CRMOs toward other ends. One interviewee described the New Left as "parasites" who would use evacuee mothers as tools for their orugu, taking advantage of their vulnerability. One interpretation was that the New Left used CRMOs to collect funds and donations or to recruit new members. Another is that the New Left provided resources (financial as well as human) to help establish and sustain some (but probably extremely few, if any) CRMOs. I do not have evidence either way, and I did not seek to probe the matter further.

The point that is most relevant for this book is the fact that the stigma of the radical groups is real for some people involved in CRMOs. Several key people in the CRMO network were highly concerned about what they saw as the infiltration of the CRMOs by the radical Left. They pointed out that any association with the radical Left would mark them as extremists, sever their relationships with foundations for those that had them, and expose them to the internal politics of the radical Left, which has a history of violence. The CRMOs' desire to be seen as apolitical comes partially from their perception of a direct threat of the damage they might suffer by being seen as "professional activists," who are embodied in the New Left.

In contemporary Japan, the legitimate space of a citizen is extremely small. Already, a good citizen is constructed as not involved in confrontational politics, as the history of the failed 1960s movements stigmatized the image of social movements. Furthermore, the radical groups paradoxically have facilitated the proregime discourse of the antinuclear movement as akin to a terrorist movement that regular citizens should stay away from. For CRMOs, the extremists' encroachment was real and present, threatening their reputation and stability. While CRMOs draw their legitimacy from being "citizen" organizations, this legitimacy is precarious and depends upon delicate maneuvering.

The Neoliberal Citizen in Citizen Science

The desire of CRMOs to avoid politics or at least to seem to avoid politics is not only because of the fear of being stigmatized for extremism. As in other cases of acute disaster, post-Fukushima Japan was a period in which national unity became a paramount theme (Okada 2012). Disaster studies scholars have noted how disasters result in social schisms (Freudenburg and Pastor 2005), but also in what has been called "therapeutic community," in which strong social ties develop (Barton 1969). Many people were moved by the scale of human tragedy, and volunteerism surged. Appearing to be politicized, because it is equated with being divisive, went against the postdisaster discourse that emphasized charity, volunteerism, and unity.

The avoidance of politics needs to be understood in relation to neo-liberalization as well. Neoliberalism can be considered an instance of a technology of the self, a mode of governmentality that exerts power by shaping one's subjectivity (Foucault 1979). Neoliberalism as articulated since the 1990s in many developed countries has reshaped the relationship between civil society and the state, and the concept of the citizen itself. A particular neoliberal citizen-subject has emerged, who is to be self-reliant and collaborative with the state, but not to oppose or challenge the existing political, social, and economic orders.

Instead of becoming radical activists, citizens are encouraged to join nongovernmental organizations (NGOs) that work with the government to provide necessary services to their fellows. Many countries that have been touched by neoliberal policy and discourses have observed a concomitant growth in NGOs. Dubbed a "shadow state" (Wolch 1990) that provides basic services that were hitherto accounted for by the state, NGOs started to work with, not against, the governments, often compelled to do so by the stark resource deprivation in communities that has resulted from neoliberal cuts. As Rebecca Dolhinow pointed out in her study of local (and female-led) NGOs in the Mexico-US border area, citizens were encouraged to be active in the community and improve the livelihood of the public, but discouraged from "creating progressive social change that challenges the systems of power that marginalize them" (2014, 143). The paradox is that while these NGOs help address the needs of impoverished communities, they simultaneously reinforce neoliberal logic and suppress radical forms of collective mobilization. The spheres of activity for citizens are now composed primarily of the market and civil society, while excluding activism. As sociologist J. Kennelly observed, the discourse tends to "neglect activism as an element of citizenship" (2009, 134).

The proliferation of NGOs is linked to a particular conceptualization of citizens as responsible for themselves. As Aihwa Ong observed with the concept of subjectification, neoliberalism installs "various regulatory regimes that govern the conduct of citizens" (1996, 738). Neoliberal citizens are those "individuals who do not need to be governed by others, but will govern themselves, master themselves, care for themselves" (Rose 1993, 285). Such neoliberal molding of the citizen has significant impacts on collective mobilization. As Wendy Brown suggests, neoliberalism "reduces political citizenship to an unprecedented degree of political passivity and complacency" because "a fully realized neoliberal citizenry would be the opposite of public-minded; indeed, it would barely exist as a public. The body politic ceases to be a body but is rather a group of individual entrepreneurs and consumers" (2005, 43, 44). Such a process of subjectification similarly has a strong impact on social mobilizations, and it tends to result in their demobilization and deradicalization (see, for instance, Dolhinow 2014).

Science is an ideal tool to perform such helpful and resourceful citizenhood. It is also usually understood as a realm with a logic different from that of politics. While science and technology studies (STS) has pointed out that science is always political, the opposite framing, which counterposes science and politics, is usually common and was ubiquitous in the interviews that I conducted with CRMO members. The boundary drawing between science and politics by citizen scientists was clear in the way responses to my questions about policy relevance and broader antinuclear movements were usually followed by some variation of "*but* our focus is good testing." The technical matter—testing—was constructed as the primary activity of the CRMO and the opposite of politics. Along the cultural boundary between scientists/science and laypeople/politics, CRMOs locate themselves on the side of the former. Many CRMOs emphasized that their core mission was to do testing well, not to push for policy change or social transformation. For instance, one CRMO in the southern region touted having a "scientist" as a member, and said its focus was on "attentive testing" (*teineina sokutei*). When I asked about their political activism, my interviewee said, "We devote ourselves totally to testing" (*sokutei ni tessuru*). "Attentive," "solid" (*shikkarishita*), and "properly" (*kichinto*) are words CRMOs often use to describe the testing they do as their self-defined mission. Testing is portrayed as a neutral action that is divorced from politics, and doing it well is the raison d'être of CRMOs.

Their self-portrayal as citizen scientists who do attentive and solid testing situates science as the polar opposite of politics. Resonating with the neoliberal citizen's codification of a citizen as practical, productive, and collaborative, this kind of citizen scientist shies away from politics and concentrates on practical and solution-oriented activities. Science helps people perform being citizens in the narrowly understood sense that fits within the neoliberal framework. This delimited citizen finds an appropriate refuge in what is considered scientific activity when oppositional politics is seen as inappropriate or unproductive for citizens. People perform being citizens by way of doing technical scientific actions, authenticating the activity of testing as a proper program for citizens.

At the same time, the notion of the citizen is an enabling symbol in doing science. Perhaps nowhere so much as in post-Fukushima Japan has the need been felt for citizens to be brought into science, as the accident resulted in a significant loss of credibility of scientific experts. It became clear to many citizens that many nuclear experts constituted a critical part of the infamous nuclear village, having a cozy relationship with pronuclear bureaucrats and the nuclear industry. The nuclear disaster damaged the legitimacy of their authority, and the scientists came to be seen as a crucial part of the problem rather than the solution. Often dubbed *goyōgakusha* or academic flunkies used by the authorities, nuclear experts were critiqued for collaborating with those in power to promote nuclear energy, underplaying the risks of nuclear reactors and the health impacts of radiation. Hence, it is not a coincidence that the self-description of CRMOs is citizen organizations. Although CRMO is my term, many identify themselves as citizen organizations, and use the term *shimin* (citizens) in their names. More than thirty out of the seventy-four CRMOs I know of have "citizen" in their names, indicating a conscious effort to identify themselves not only as science-related organizations, but as citizen organizations.

There is a double movement in post-Fukushima citizen science: On the one hand, citizens have become the torchbearers for a neutral and credible science. "Citizen" conjures a feeling of authenticity and neutrality, an identity that strikes a chord with many people who have lost their trust in mainstream scientists and the government. On the other hand, the space for citizens is increasingly constrained to conform to the neoliberal ideal of productive and personally responsible citizens. Citizen science therefore means a move to rescue science from politics, and also a move to rescue citizens from politics.

Measuring on the Margin

In the increasingly narrow space for legitimate citizens, doing science by way of measuring radiation is a performance of being a citizen, conjuring a scientific and technical image as apolitical and neutral. Sharing the aura of science helps people to perform being legitimate citizens, who are solution-oriented, moderate, and agreeable.

But CRMOs have not become completely depoliticized by withdrawing into science. I suggest that the traditional view of politics is inadequate for understanding the space of citizen science in contemporary society. The social movement literature would privilege oppositional politics, in which citizens confront the elite with explicit social change objectives and policy-relevant activities on a sustained basis. It is hard to find these characteristics in CRMOs. They concentrate on scientific activities with the objective of accumulating data rather than effecting political change, and they rarely seem to have a plan for long-term organizational maintenance. Even if CRMOs might not count as social movement organizations, however, their complete domestication is not necessarily the only possible end result. In order to understand the energy and passion that people have invested in CRMOs, we need to see politics differently from the view that privileges electoral and policy dimensions. For CRMOs, data collecting by measuring already constitutes a political action, rather than only being a means to something bigger—traditional politics with a capital P. In a climate that significantly limits the oppositional framing of issues and people, citizen science is ascribed political undertones.

Samuels (2013a, 132) observed, as mentioned in the introduction, that people in Japan seemed more "concerned than outraged" in the wake of the nuclear accidents. The choice to organize CRMOs rather than, say, volunteering for the Green Party or organizing sit-ins might seem at first glance to express nothing more than concern. Yet their outrage might have been channeled into testing as a means for politics. Although CRMOs apparently do little more than run detectors, my interviews suggested that the people involved in them attach complex meanings to testing that go beyond the simple operation of a detector. The testing done by CRMOs can be described as measuring on the margin. By this term, I refer to a praxis by subaltern groups of enacting an alternative reality by way of technical measurement, an instance of ontological politics where plural realities constitute the heart of social contestation (Woolgar and Lezaun 2013b). Testing describes a certain reality—"this peach is contaminated at 10 Bq/kg"—that was not known before the measurement. Testing makes the invisible visible, enabling a different kind of conversation to take place, which might have consequences for policies.

Feminists have particularly noted the importance of making the invisible visible by way of scientific practice. Historian Michelle Murphy (2006) examined women's endeavors to give shape to what is now known as toxic building syndrome. Women who suffered from it had to do something to give shape to the invisible, to transform unarticulable experiences into a form that was invested with more social power. With various strategies, these women successfully made the previously invisible and politically neglected both visible and politically articulable. One of the strategies was to conduct a survey. The survey was able to turn "'counter-knowledge' into evidence" that was quantifiable and "more palatable to the bureaucrat" (73). The transformation of experience to data with the use of a survey was necessary to counter what Murphy calls the regime of perceptibility. It is with this kind of anticipation of an increased ability to enact a different reality that measuring on the margin is conducted.

But not all testing is subversive, even when it is done on the margins of society. Consider the example of ETHOS (chapter 2). ETHOS promotes testing by local residents as part of the praxis of so-called practical radiological protection culture (PRPC). Testing as part of PRPC bears a strongly conservative meaning. When ETHOS emphasizes the need to measure internal and external radiation, it is as "self-help protective actions" that aim "at the characterisation of their own radiological situation" for "adapting their way of life accordingly to reduce their exposure" (Lochard et al. 2009, 12). Under the strong influence of neoliberal pressure for personal responsibility, testing can be refashioned into a means for individuals to take responsibility for managing their exposure levels rather than holding the government and the nuclear industry accountable for contamination.

My examination of CRMOs suggests multiple ways in which the testing that they do becomes subversive. First, people test collectively and/or share their results with others. Like a thermometer or a scale, a radiation detector can be a completely private gadget for personal use. In contrast, the CRMOs are a means for communal measurement. The collective aspect of measuring is consciously chosen, and this becomes obvious in the cases of the several CRMOs that were started by individuals who bought detectors to test food for their own families. They started accepting other people's requests to test food, and now they operate as CRMOs. In some other cases, the testing is done by one person, but the spirit is always communal. People tweet the measuring results; they use listservs to exchange results and tips for testing. Simply testing food by yourself, withdrawing from the social world, is not subversive. But testing together becomes an act of sharing a particular view of reality.

Second, testing becomes subversive when it exposes the mistakes and blind spots in the official testing programs. The CRMOs feel that their sheer existence as a third eye is important to warn the government that they are being watched. In some cases, this watchdog function is more concrete. For instance, CRMO members in the Tokyo metropolitan area talked about how they found a mistake in the government data. The municipality-operated program in Tokyo tested barley far below the government standard of 100 Bq/kg, but when the CRMO retested the same sample, they found that it actually exceeded it. With those data in hand, the CRMO members demanded that the municipality test food more accurately.[8]

Another kind of subversiveness lies in the fact that CRMOs often test for contamination to contradict the version of reality put forth by the government. For instance, some CRMOs look for food that is likely to be contaminated. While the usual samples tested at CRMOs are brought in by customers, many CRMOs also include samples of their choice. Several CRMOs that I interviewed tended to test food that was likely to be contaminated—such as wild game and foraged mushrooms and herbs, which are already known from government data to be highly contaminated. In one CRMO in western Japan, a staff member talked about how he went to multiple supermarkets looking for vegetables and fruits from the northeastern region to be measured. These efforts would be simply perverse if the CRMOs' function was only to help citizens avoid contaminated food. But their actions need to be situated in relation to how measuring on the margin is about contradicting the authorized version of reality.

If CRMOs can find some contamination, even below government standards, the contamination becomes reality, so to speak. The unit of concentration, the becquerel, has become a verb. Members of CRMOs talk about how a thing "becquereled" or not (*bekureta/bekurenai*) to indicate finding or not finding any concentration of cesium in a sample. To test is "to becquerel," an action to help inscribe the reality of the existence of cesium somewhere that it might not otherwise have been recognized as existing.

Some CRMOs seek unique means of testing. For instance, a CRMO in the northeastern region suspected, like many citizens, that manufacturers were using contaminated food by diluting it to keep the concentrations of contamination lower than the government standards. Processed food became particularly worrisome, and they decided to measure yogurt, as milk was frequently found contaminated, particularly in 2011. Since it was likely diluted, they reasoned that they needed to have a condensed sample. They bought more than a dozen containers of yogurt, tried to dry it by spreading it in a dryer and baking it for an extended period of time, and then made a sample by crushing the dried sheets of yogurt. The reason this CRMO invested this amount of labor cannot be fully understood without realizing that the point was to prove that the yogurt becquereled. The testing indeed found approximately 0.97 Bq/kg.[9] From the perspective of the government, this kind of data would be considered irrelevant as no one would consume that much yogurt in such a condensed form, and the number is far below the government standard of 100 Bq/kg. But the CRMO's blog entry concluded, "Surely, it becquereled!" with apparent satisfaction at confirming their suspicion that contaminated food was still circulating (Bekuredenegana 2014).

It is important to underscore here that testing in the center is no less culpable for producing a particular kind of reality. If the above description gives the impression that measuring on the margin is somehow skewed and deliberately tampers with the evidence to produce a certain result, measuring in the center is no different. For instance, it was widely rumored that the air contamination data from monitoring posts run by the government tended to show much lower levels of contamination than the data from nongovernment monitoring posts, because the areas surrounding the government posts were decontaminated meticulously.

The level of contamination of tea and dried shiitake mushrooms and herbs is another example. For the government's testing processes, the samples are not in dried form, but in the form in which the items would actually be consumed. According to the Ministry of Agriculture, tea leaves need to be soaked in water thirty times the weight of the tea for sixty minutes. Dried shiitake mushrooms need to be soaked in water before being tested, or the result obtained with the sample in dried form must be divided by a specific conversion rate (the rate was set at 5.7, so dried mushrooms with a level of 523 Bq/kg would be listed as having 91.7 Bq/kg). The justification for these procedures is that the contamination level would be close to that of the food when people consume it, but critics point out that the dilution would result in lower levels of cesium.

If neoliberal subjectivity conjures a rationally calculating citizen who is individualistic and self-centered, measuring on the margin is done by people in a different kind of affective state. Measuring on the margin is not a solitary achievement of a rationally self-interested individual, nor an act of personal responsibility mandated by neoliberal governmentality. It is rooted in a sense of shared interest that is not utilitarian. My interviews with CRMOs highlighted the multiple meanings of testing to those who work there. Of course, the typical narrative started with how they wanted to ensure the safety of the food they were eating and feeding to their family members. But that was only part of it, and many of the people I interviewed talked about their sense of connection to other people and their desire to do something for others. When I was at a CRMO in western Japan, for instance, I met a group of volunteers. They were all well-dressed middle-aged women. I asked one of them, Takeshita-san, a married woman in her forties, about her work at the CRMO. She said she had been totally apolitical, and thought that people involved in antinuclear issues were rather different from her. When I asked her whether she was doing social activism through her CRMO, she looked unsure of what to say but replied, "I am not sure about the term social activism [*shimin katsudō*]. I just . . . just wanted to know the reality of the food. And I wanted to do something after the accident for people in the affected areas. For me, it is a way *to be with* [*yorisou*] Fukushima." By saying that her motivation for testing was "to be with Fukushima," she underscored that testing was more than the act of running a detector, but rather praxis imbued with emotional symbolism of solidarity and sympathy.

In summary, testing by CRMOs is not simply about running a detector and getting a printout of estimates. They provide data that support a counternarrative to the official discourse that paints a picture in which cesium does not exist in food on the market. By enacting a different reality—however low the contamination might be, and even when the official scientific wisdom would say that such a low level does not matter—they are able to enact a profound shift in reality, from the nonexistence of contamination to its existence.

Conclusion

Citizen science is often celebrated as a democratization of science and the inclusion of laypeople as legitimate partners in the making of knowledge. Questioning such an uncritical espousal of citizen science, this chapter has analyzed CRMOs as a unique lens through which complicated understandings of the political contribution of citizen science can emerge.

The examination of CRMOs in this chapter shows how citizen scientists are constrained by neoliberal subjectification that renders citizen-subjects into responsible and resourceful beings. The strong scientization of policy making, combined with such neoliberal influences, makes science an alluring way to perform the ideal citizen-subject, while at the same time pulling citizen scientists away from politics. The impressive proliferation of CRMOs after the Fukushima nuclear disaster is paradoxically a reflection of the increasingly restricted space of the citizen in Japan, as much as of the actual need to know if food is contaminated.

But at the same time, despite the mandate for neoliberal citizens to remain apolitical, testing provides a subtle means to be politically engaged. While many CRMOs have a professed policy of being nonpolitical, they cannot be accurately described as apolitical and domesticated. Their original motivation was concern about food safety, despite the government dictum that instructed citizens not to worry about it. They take the form of collective action—although testing one's food alone is possible, they opt to do it with and for others. The CRMOs also try various strategies to reveal contamination and alert the public.

I use the concept "measuring on the margin" to understand this jarring sense of politics in the technical praxis of citizen scientists. Seemingly simply technical, measuring the level of cesium in food garners such passion and commitment from citizens because it has the potential to enact a different reality of the postdisaster world. Testing can itself be a form of politics, legitimating a different understanding of reality than the government-sanctioned one.

Measuring on the margin is not always politically efficacious, but sometimes it is, often by producing a number that can do the work, so to speak. Like Dipesh Chakrabarty's (1992) ghosts in India who do the job of speaking on behalf of people, numbers rather than particular individuals or groups can enter a political conversation. Test results can play a highly political role, while letting CRMOs act simply as a conduit of data. By deferring agency to the results, that seemingly unbiased thing, data, can talk by itself. In a context where politics is stigmatized, this creation of a number-subject is a useful political strategy. Of course, the number cannot be just any number. Its pedigree is important; whether it is produced by testing done by the Communist Party or by a CRMO shapes how the number is responded to. The conscious naming of CRMOs as citizen organizations therefore helps to authenticate the numbers they produce as trustworthy political subjects.

It is for this reason that counteraction by the elites has often attacked the pedigree of the numbers. This dynamic became obvious, for instance, when the Ministry of Education and Technology issued instructions saying that measurement by scintillation detectors—which are used by the vast majority of CRMOs—had a problem of precision and so germanium semiconductor detectors should be used instead (Inoue 2012). The latter are much more expensive than scintillators, and most CRMOs cannot afford them. By saying that the germanium detector unequivocally provides the truth and the scintillation detector does not, this government move worked to delegitimize the bulk of testing done by CRMOs.

Within STS, various strands of literature have tried to understand different ways of doing politics.[10] As political scientist and STS scholar Mark Brown (2009) argued in his book *Science in Democracy*, if scientific representation is as political as political representation, then testing is about representing reality in order to enact a particular materiality of the world. Testing makes certain things become recognizable, laying a basis for legitimating a particular understanding of the world (Daston 2000, 2008; Hacking 2002).[11]

Why people show such great satisfaction, while engaged in the seemingly dull and routinized procedure of testing at CRMOs, is related to the potential of measuring on the margin to constitute a different kind of reality that might jolt the existing social and technical orders. Ignorance or absence of knowledge has a close resemblance to secrets—hence the pleasure of discovering it (High, Kelly, and Mair 2012). Measuring radiation and becquerels can be about exposing a "public secret" (Taussig 1999), what is generally known but should not be articulated. A story that one interviewee at a CRMO shared seemed initially tangential to my research, but now its importance is clear. At the end of a long interview, he mentioned that he took multiple trips to the areas surrounding the troubled reactors. He would bring his Geiger counter and collect samples of soil to be tested later at the lab. The way he described the trips was filled with excitement and curiosity, like a hunter looking for charismatic animals. It would seem paradoxical for someone who was concerned with food contamination to visit contaminated places, if one of the points of testing is to avoid radiation exposure. Yet what testing can entail seems close to the discovery of deeply hidden secrets. Like getting a peek into the workings of infrastructure and systems that are naturalized and taken for granted (Star 1999), testing can be a thrill, an adventure into a hitherto hidden world.

This chapter is motivated by the question of why science, not radical politics, was chosen by citizens as a way to counter food policing by the authorities and experts. Measuring on the margin obviously gets at the heart of a matter of contention—whether food is contaminated or not and how badly. But it is also a product of the scientism and neoliberalization that make citizen science a helpful way to perform the legitimate citizen-subject.

CRMOs are not an immature form of social movement organization. They are, rather, a form that is necessitated by the scientization of politics as well as the neoliberalization of the citizen in citizen science. Doing science is a way to align with the image of the citizen that is agreeable and accepted. But measuring on the margin can also be a tool of accountability and investigation into the conduct of the pronuclear forces. People measure with affect, sometimes finding a thrill in their ability to enact a reality that contradicts the elite's version. Despite the lack of obvious forms of mobilization, measuring can be mobilizing, the mobilizing of a certain sociality that does matter.

FIVE

The Temporality of Contaminants

After the Fukushima nuclear accident, CRMOs started up in many places across Japan and garnered strong support from ordinary citizens. But the existence of CRMOs is insecure. They spread rapidly after the accident, and they have tested a large number of food samples. But many of them operate on a shoestring budget and depend upon the small fees they charge customers who bring in food to be tested. Three years had passed since the accident by the time I conducted most of the interviews with CRMOs for this book, and there was already a decline in the number of citizens bringing in food to be tested; many CRMOs seemed to be suffering from financial difficulties, and some had been forced to shut down.

The precariousness of CRMOs might be considered a logical consequence of the decline in the discovery of contaminated food as time passed following the nuclear accident. However, this chapter critically examines the notion that CRMOs were obsolete by 2014. The number of active CRMOs seems to have declined not only because the initial panic has subsided and fewer cases of contamination are being discovered but due to a broader social dynamics. I point to the intersecting influences of gender ideologies, neoliberalism, and scientism.

Two issues are highlighted in this chapter. First, the precarious existence of CRMOs suggests the growing burden on neoliberal citizens who have shouldered an increasing amount of care work in an atmosphere of shrinking social protection, leaving people ever less time for political and communal activities. Globally, neoliberalism has exacerbated the gap between the rich and the poor, and those on the economic margins face tougher economic situations with shrinking social safety nets, even in a country like Japan, which is much more of a welfare state than countries like the United States. Pressed to meet their basic economic needs, more and more people feel they rarely have time and energy to invest in noneconomic activities. It was inevitable that food contamination would become less pressing as the years have passed since 2011, and some people involved in CRMOs have moved on to respond to other pressing needs in their lives. This is particularly true of women, not only because they have often served as the leaders and staff members of CRMOs, but also because care work is culturally codified as female. There is a vast feminist literature on how care work has historically been feminized. It is women who typically shoulder unpaid care work within family. Care work as paid work has historically also been a highly feminized sector that tends to face what is called the care penalty—meager pay and few benefits with little job security or mobility (England 1994; Glenn 2000; Weigt 2006). Furthermore, neoliberal cuts in social services often result in increasing care burdens (often unpaid) for women. Women tend to shoulder most of the responsibility of caring for others, and they constantly face one care need after another, from children, other family members, the elderly, and the sick.

Neoliberalism also has had a significant influence on how contaminants—radioactive materials—are viewed in post-Fukushima Japan. In particular, I want to draw attention to the temporality of contaminants and how neoliberalism's anticipatory tendency influences it. Scholars have argued that neoliberalism requires and normalizes a particular kind of psychological state that Adams, Murphy, and Clarke (2009, 247) called a "regime of anticipation," which propels individuals, communities, and nations to look forward to the future as pregnant with opportunities. This anticipatory outlook helps frame radiation as the product of a single, contained event, which belongs increasingly to the past. Radioactive materials have been quickly rendered an antiquated concern that is unwelcome in a postaccident nation that is looking to rebuild and to heal its fractured confidence in itself. This temporality has helped construct the obsoleteness of CRMOs, while legitimizing a vision of the future that touts dealing with contaminants smartly—meaning through technical and scientific means, rather than political and social ones.

The chapter's findings have significant implications for theories of citizen science. First, citizen science is often carried out by women; their increased care burden under neoliberalism makes it harder for them to engage in citizen science and to make it a tool for political activism. Citizen science therefore may become increasingly ephemeral as well as restrained under neoliberalism. The neoliberal regime of anticipation also propels citizen science toward being a short- to medium-term response to disaster situations (as laudable self-help by responsible individuals) but constrains it from branching out to long-term prevention of harm. The regime of anticipation shapes citizen science to emphasize that contaminants can be prepared for rather than prevented. Therefore, we need to carefully watch how citizen science might be directed to disaster relief and perhaps even disaster preparedness but not disaster prevention.

The Sustainability of CRMOs

As the previous chapter summarized, CRMOs began to spread in the summer of 2011 and were established across Japan. But many of them have struggled to remain open and active. The CRMOs' instability is rooted in various issues. For most of the period that I observed them, between 2011 and 2014, CRMOs did not organize or develop formal networks among themselves. One exception is the network of seven CRMOs mentioned in chapter 4, the Citizen Radiation-Measuring Stations. Another exception is Everyone's Data Site (Minna no Dēta Saito), which was initially organized by the Citizen Radiation-Measuring Stations network, several other CRMOs, and a longtime antinuclear organization, the Takagi Fund for Citizen Science. Their objective was to launch a website that consolidated data from CRMOs across the country so that citizens could log in and find relevant measuring results easily. The website was launched in September 2013 with measurement data from about twenty CRMOs, but their funding became tricky. A part of the grant used for Everyone's Data Site came from the Mitsui Environmental Fund, a corporate social responsibility (CSR) program of the trading giant, Mitsui Corporation. Some of the organizations involved in the project felt that this was akin to receiving money from the enemy, as Mitsui had been involved in exporting nuclear reactors abroad, and some CRMOs decided to withdraw from the project. Nonetheless, the project went ahead and now offers a searchable website (Minna no Data Site, http://www.minnanods.net/) based on measurement data from member CRMOs after ensuring their testing capacities are up to standard. It also started a national project to measure the contamination level of soil in 2014 with the thought that an accurate understanding of contamination would be increasingly difficult due to the shorter half-life of cesium 134.

In addition to the difficulty of horizontal networking, the problem of financing has emerged as a major challenge for many CRMOs. Most of the time, CRMOs have been funded with grassroots donations. Only one CRMO—the aforementioned one in Koganei City, founded after Chernobyl—received some help from a municipal government. In many cases, citizens solicited money from small donors to establish CRMOs; some received help from foundations and private groups, such as the Takagi Fund; DAYS Japan, the publisher of a progressive news magazine; and the Catalogue House, an alternative retailer, just to name a few. Besides the purchase of the detectors, which cost from US $10,000–$80,000, CRMOs incur various costs such as rent, supplies, and utilities. The CRMOs might be able to pay for a detector, but for most of them the operational costs are hard to cover on a sustained basis. Some CRMOs save money by using a space in an existing business, such as another nonprofit organization, a café, a restaurant, or a farm, but others that operate solely as CRMOs incur significant costs to rent space. In order to address these financial issues, many CRMOs chose a membership structure. For instance, one in Kyoto had over 200 members in 2013, each paying 4,000 yen (around US $40) as an annual fee. And many CRMOs ask their clients to pay for testing services, with prices ranging from 500 to 7,000 yen per sample.

Most CRMOs need either a substantial membership that continues paying annual fees or a large enough number of customers paying testing fees. But many CRMOs have been experiencing a decline in those numbers; fewer and fewer people come to test their food as the years pass since the accident. From 2011 to 2013, the cumulative number of samples tested by CRMOs I contacted was impressive, but many fewer samples were tested in 2013. Furthermore, municipal governments have started to offer similar testing services, usually for free. The proliferation of CRMOs and the establishment of the government programs have created price competition, forcing some organizations to reduce the fee per sample and to compete for customers.

A CRMO in the metropolitan Tokyo area, for instance, was established by a man in his forties who at the time of the accident had just been laid off because of the recession. Because his family lived in a place that was identified as a hot spot and he had an infant, he became concerned about the contamination of tap water and food. They could not relocate for various reasons, including the loan on their condo. He decided to open a CRMO, bought a detector, and rented a space. For the first two years, this CRMO had many customers, but in 2013 it was impossible for him to make a living from it. When I interviewed him in 2014, he looked distressed and was considering selling the detector or renting it to someone else, as he had to provide for his family.

The lack of organizational infrastructure for CRMOs mirrors a broader picture of the Japanese nonprofit sector. As political scientist Robert Pekkanen observed, Japanese civil society has long been characterized by a large number of small organizations that do not have paid staff and largely run on volunteer labor, unlike many Western nonprofits, which can be large and professionalized, with sustainable revenue bases such as solid membership, donations, or foundation grants (Pekkanen 2006).

Within only a few years of the accident, many CRMOs were facing difficult challenges. The financial costs of keeping a CRMO running are sometimes too large for a group of people who have often patched together their individual savings and depend upon their personal networks to collect resources just sufficient to start such a group. In addition, the number of clients who are willing to pay for measurement has tended to go down due to increased competition from government-run measurement programs as well as among CRMOs and the decrease in general interest in the topic of food contamination. And as the years pass, it is also inevitable that public interest in the topic declines. Although many CRMOs would prefer to stay open, they generally face challenges in paying their operational costs out of their shrinking revenue.

Debating the Continued Relevance of CRMOs

The decline of CRMOs would be considered a logical trend in the dominant discourse, which emphasizes that contaminants in the environment are declining as time passes since the nuclear accident. In general, the government wants the country to move on quickly, marking the triple disasters—earthquake, tsunami, and nuclear accident—as a historic event to be commemorated. But unlike the earthquake and tsunami, the nuclear accident is a particularly sticky problem for this framing as its end point is hard to pin down. Nonetheless, the government continues to try to paint a picture in which food contamination by radioactive materials was a one-shot deal; certainly unfortunate, but something that belongs to the historic and contained events of March 2011. For instance, in December 2011, in a remarkable denial of the continuing troubles at the Fukushima No. 1 nuclear power plant, Prime Minister Noda Yoshihiko declared that the accident had been "brought to a conclusion" (Cabinet Office 2011). Two years later in October 2013, when the plant was still coping with many issues, particularly the leaking of polluted water into the ocean, Prime Minister Abe Shinzo proclaimed to the international community that it was "under control" in his bid for Tokyo as an Olympic host city (Cabinet Office 2013b).

The government's news releases and public relations materials emphasize that the discovery of contaminated food has become rare. The message in 2013 was already, to quote a report by the Ministry of Health, Labor, and Welfare, that "the concentration of radioactive materials in food from the accident has decreased and is currently at an extremely low level" (2013, 30). Indeed, out of 19,657 vegetable samples tested by the Ministry of Agriculture in 2013, none exceeded the government standard (100 Bq/kg). Only twenty-eight out of more than 10 million samples of rice were contaminated above 100 Bq/kg (Ministry of Agriculture, Forestry and Fisheries 2014).[1] This kind of data helps to paint a picture of the radioactive contamination as a historic event. And in fact, already by 2014, some government officials had started to talk about easing the food standards ("Shokuhin No Hōshaseibusshitsukijyun Hijyō Ni Gimon" 2014; "Shokuhin No Hōshaseibusshitsukijyun Kanwa Kentō" 2014).

If CRMOs are considered a response to the Fukushima accident only, then their quick decline is to be expected. The most obvious role of CRMOs was to provide testing services to citizens immediately after the accident when the government testing services were not open to the public and the patterns of contamination were unknown. However, CRMOs have other roles as well, such as acting as watchdogs on the government's testing activities and providing spaces for sharing concerns, exchanging information, and training citizens. The view that sees only a short-term use for CRMOs fails to recognize their multiple functions.

One important role that CRMOs took on was that of watchdog vis-à-vis the authorities, as they keep a close eye on government-released data at both national and local levels. Chapter 4 mentioned one example of how a CRMO found an error in a municipal government's data on food contamination levels. This kind of watchdog role continued to be relevant even after the government testing programs became established, especially given the long history of data falsification and minimization of risk by the authorities and the nuclear industry in Japan (Koide 2011).[2]

The CRMOs also have provided a space for citizens to share concerns, to gather, and to exchange information. For instance, a CRMO run by a consortium of Christian churches recognized that citizens need not only the data results from food testing, but someone to talk to about their concerns about food contamination and health risks. They decided to hire a staff member experienced in counseling. This CRMO also prepared a comfortable space with a cozy sofa and plenty of room. While having a counseling professional on staff is unusual among CRMOs, many of them do envision their role to include not only measuring the level of food contamination but also making a space for citizens to share their worries and concerns. This function is important, as one of my interviewees put it, because "people cannot do it outside." Many of the CRMO staff members I interviewed talked about how people came and confessed their relief at being able to admit they were worried about radiation contamination, because the government and scientists emphasized the safety of food and criticized people who questioned it. Kataoka Terumi, a woman who established a CRMO in Fukushima, wrote that one of its important functions was to provide *shaberiba* (a place to chat), saying, "The people who come are people who could not say what they felt. They felt that they were strange because of worrying too much. But they can come [to the CRMO] and share their feelings, and they can confirm that, ah, I am not a strange person, my feeling is not wrong" (Kataoka 2012, 44). She herself felt the pressure not to talk about food contamination. She recalled how she had asked herself, "Is my worry only an overreaction? Am I a crazy person who is too concerned with radiation? My individual concern was growing but I could not talk about it. If I talked about it, I was told, you are strange, overly cautious, or I felt like I was going to be told something like that" (35–36). As anthropologist David Slater and his collaborators observed, postaccident Japan saw a widespread "medicalizing discourse that cast radiation fears as the result of individual pathology" and that particularly targeted women (Slater, Morioka, and Danzuka 2014, 503). The CRMOs function as a space for sharing concerns without having to fear being labeled "crazy" and "overly nervous" (Slater, Morioka, and Danzuka 2014, 505). As Nicolas Sternsdorff-Cisterna writes, food safety is not only about technical parameters (*anzen* in Japanese) but also about feeling safe (*anshin* in Japanese) which is aided by collective meaning making in one's social network. The CRMOs provide a space where people can create what he calls "affective networks of trust" (Sternsdorff-Cisterna 2015, 2).

In addition, CRMOs generally provide more information and explanation to the clients who bring in food to be tested than the government-run testing programs do. When I went to a testing program operated by the City of Fukushima, for instance, I saw people dropping off an item to be measured and coming back in thirty minutes or so to receive a printout. I obtained a sample printout that read, "Dear Mr. X. In regard to your request for a measurement of radioactive materials on X/X/2013, it is as follows," with a simple table of three rows indicating densities of cesium 134, cesium 137, and the total of the two. It said nothing about the process of measurement except for the name of the detector (Belarus ATOMTEX Co. NaI Scintillator). It had no graph showing a spectrum of radionuclides, which is critical to interpreting estimates of radioactive materials. In an interview, a program staff member talked about how he had actually requested the manufacturer of the software for the detector to simplify the letter's format by removing the spectrum. He said that it would "confuse middle-aged men and women [*ojichan obachan*]."

In contrast, most CRMOs provide much more detailed information. Part of the reason is that they want to demonstrate the validity of their results by showing the details of the test. Therefore, it is common for them to attach a copy of the spectrum produced by the test. On a deeper level, however, they trust that even regular citizens—even ojichan obachan—can understand and should be informed of the details (and the necessary ambiguity) of the radiation data. When I asked CRMO staff people in interviews how long they took to explain the results, many said that it could take a long time particularly early on when people had little information and knowledge about the radiation measurement, and they often engaged in extended conversation with clients. Many of them had a folder that contained information to be shown to clients to explain how the detector worked, how to read the spectrum, and recent test results to show trends in food contamination. The government testing programs simply focus on giving the results; hence the counseling and educational function of CRMOs still plays an important role, even with the current availability of government programs.

Also, CRMOs can be considered as enhancing the capacity of the society as a whole to respond to the next nuclear disaster. They not only educate general citizens but provide opportunities for their staff members to hone their skills in radiation detection and measurement. CRMOs utilize various means such as workshops, e-mail exchanges, and listservs to improve their measuring skills. For instance, six CRMOs in the western region formed a network and meet once every two months to discuss testing skills. In one of the meetings that I attended, staff members from the six CRMOs shared what they felt to be *kininaru dēta* (data that is worrisome) from recent months. They discussed how to deal with challenges in producing good measurements. Furthermore, some CRMOs have worked with detector manufacturers to improve their ability to provide solid measurements. Both detectors and software come with various bugs, and many CRMOs have consulted with the manufacturers or the analytical software developers to increase the ease of operation and precision of measurement.[3]

Many interviewees pointed out that the half-life of cesium 137 is more than thirty years and so, ideally, CRMOs should exist for that long. Furthermore, many of them pointed out that Japan had the third most nuclear power plants in the world (forty-eight commercial plants) and although all of them were closed after the Fukushima accident, the government and the industry are on the path to resuming their operation. Many Japanese reactors are old; seventeen of the plants were built more than thirty years ago. Aging power plants are more accident prone, as radioactivity damages the infrastructure of the plants even during normal operation. Given the highly complex nature of nuclear power plants, small accidents are not uncommon, and some of them can result in serious releases of radioactivity into the environment. In addition, Japan is also one of the most earthquake-prone countries. Although the nuclear industry argues that the nuclear power plants are "designed to withstand earthquakes, and in the event of major earth movement, to shut down safely" (World Nuclear Association 2014), the Fukushima case raises significant doubts about such assurances. The CRMOs could be considered part of a necessary safety structure in the context of Japan's highly volatile and risk-prone nuclear situation; they could be seen as integral to food security in an age when radioactive materials are already present in the environment and/or in areas where nuclear reactors are in operation.

It should also be pointed out that because food systems are increasingly delocalized, having CRMOs in various places in a nation would be helpful. While land contamination might be localized to the vicinity of a particular nuclear reactor, the Japanese food system is integrated in a way that makes it difficult to localize the distribution of contaminated foods. Rather than self-sufficiency within a particular locale, trading among different regions, for instance, of vegetables, has increased. Since the 1960s, government policies have directed many agricultural regions to concentrate on a particular signature product so as to take advantage of scale of production and niche marketing (Araki 2002; Takayanagi 2006). Consumers are increasingly buying foods from supermarkets and convenience stores rather than from small neighborhood stores (Satō 2011). Regional, national, and global retail chains tend to directly procure foods from producers, giving an advantage to relatively large-scale producing regions that can meet the quality and volume requirements (Konosu 2004). Such extralocal circulation of foods coexists with more localized channels such as the farmers' markets and organic share farms promoted by local food movements that have gained popularity in recent years (Kimura and Nishiyama 2008).

One might argue that the decline in CRMOs is a logical consequence of the now-sufficient testing services offered by the government as well as the rapid decline in contamination and corresponding declining public concern about the issue. But such a view neglects the fact that the role of CRMOs encompasses not only the emergency testing of food samples but also the verification of government data, education and training of laypeople, and building of a social network where one can interpret safety issues collectively. Another perspective would also argue that as long as there are nuclear reactors in Japan, the next nuclear disaster ought to be expected; hence CRMOs ought to be considered a feature of the normal governance of food safety in a society that is not immune from radiation threats. But the rapid decline in public interest is a hard reality that CRMOs had to face only three years after the Fukushima nuclear accident.

The Temporal Politics of Contaminants

In the opening speech of the 2014 parliamentary session, Prime Minister Abe Shinzo described the situation of the areas affected by the triple disasters with an undeterred optimism for the future: "Off the coast of

Fukushima, floating offshore wind farms will have started their operations. In Miyagi, sweet strawberries will be cultivated in large-scale greenhouses. . . . We also now find rice paddies where planting has been resumed, fishing ports overflowing with the joy of the day's catches, and public housing filled with families' happy faces. We will make Tōhoku, which lost so much in the earthquake disaster, a pioneering region where the world's most advanced new technologies will put forth buds" (Abe 2014). Here is a vision for the food system in the affected region, filled with upgraded seafood processing ventures and high-tech strawberry factories. But conspicuously absent from this imaginary Tōhoku are radioactive materials in the soil and ocean. The absence of radioactive contaminants in Abe's vision of the future is even stranger when one considers that some radionuclides are known to remain in the environment for decades. Yet contaminants have no place in this vision except as an artifact belonging to the past. They caused a huge loss; but on the path to becoming a "pioneering region where the world's most advanced new technologies will put forth buds," they are an obstacle already almost overcome.

How do we explain this glaring absence of contaminants? While it is possible to consider it simply a politician's wishful forgetfulness of anything negative, I argue that Abe's speech was also a reflection of an affective work of neoliberalism that attempts "to more closely align emotions with imperatives of the market and the state" (Ramos-Zayas 2012, 6). Such an emotional state is an important element in the neoliberal regime of anticipation, where "anticipation has become a common, lived affect-state of daily life, shaping regimes of self, health and spirituality" (Adams, Murphy, and Clarke 2009, 247). The regime of anticipation summons a strong aspirationalism with an emphasis on hope for the future and excited entrepreneurism in anticipation of a coming payoff.

This anticipatory regime influences how contaminants are socially presented as well, particularly in relation to their temporality. Once Japan emerged from the state of emergency in the immediate aftermath of the accident, the impacts of radioactive materials here and now were less and less discussed. Rather than being portrayed as something still in the environment, radioactive contaminants are now seen as already contained and belonging to the past. Because the anticipatory mode's affective requirement is to be in an "excited, forward looking subjective condition" (Adams, Murphy, and Clarke 2009, 247), any talk about contaminants in the present is condemned as annoying negativity that is not productive and constructive. Postdisaster nationalism raised the stakes on the absence of contaminants, as the nuclear accident further tarnished the image of Japan in the international community when Japan was already struggling with its national branding (see Hymans 2010) in the shadow of both China and a prolonged recession (McGray 2009; Valaskivi 2013). Even mentioning contamination goes against the national yearning for a positive spin and the dictum that good Japanese citizens are forward looking and positive thinking, all sharing the national aspiration for the "rebirth" of the nation (Samuels 2013b, 2), not unlike its rebirth after the devastation of World War II.

Of course, neoliberal anticipation conjures both risk and future disasters, not only hope and aspiration. Scholars have noted how the concept of disaster preparedness has become popular among policy makers since the 1990s. While the preparedness approach seems to be a welcome trend toward prevention in contrast to only responses after the fact, critical analyses have pointed out that it is also a product of the neoliberal turn in its emphasis on self-defense and self-help. As Clare Jen examined in regard to the global severe acute respiratory syndrome (SARS) scare, the responsibility of protection is transferred from the government to citizens who are then prompted to purchase self-protective services and gear. Women and other marginalized groups are often highlighted as the harbingers of risk and contaminants, while the systemic issues that result in their vulnerability are not addressed (Jen 2013). The preparedness approach takes the existing social structure as a given, although it is often constitutive of vulnerability to risk and disasters. Instead, the preparedness approach redirects people to focus on "an artificial and depoliticized form of adaptive capacity that does not threaten neoliberal order" (Grove 2014, 240). In this way, the call for future preparedness replaces the call for prevention. As Adams, Murphy, and Clarke wrote, the neoliberal approach focuses more on "generating new and better means of dealing with inevitable disasters than actually preventing them" (2009, 258).

Preparedness is also constructed in a peculiar manner—it has to be "smart" in its technical solutions. Take the strawberries that Abe mentioned. Produced with a postdisaster subsidy from a government project called Advanced Technology Development for Reconstructing Food-Producing Areas, the strawberries embody the smart solutions to the food safety threats posed by the nuclear accident. Here, radiation contamination is addressed by a version of the increasingly popular vegetable or fruit factories, in which vegetables and fruits are produced indoors in a controlled environment so as to avoid radiation and other airborne pollutants. These strawberries in their high-tech vinyl houses are not so much grown as manufactured; rather than living in soil, they depend on a comprehensive aquaponic system (provided by a corporation). The strawberries are smart in two senses: First, they are "radiation proof" because their indoor environment is completely controlled; and second, they are the embodiment of value added, as a branded product rather than an undifferentiated agricultural commodity. This new, trademarked brand of strawberries, Migakiichigo (shining strawberries), is now sold at upscale department stores aiming at high-end consumers.[4] The smart strawberries embody the government and corporate vision for the future of Japanese agriculture. Even before the accident, the government considered the Japanese agricultural sector unsophisticated and in need of radical restructuring, and had advocated what it called "strong agriculture" as a solution. As in the United States after Hurricane Katrina, the disaster provided fertile ground to further push the neoliberal agenda.

Disaster studies scholars have pointed out that policies tend to take the position of disaster exceptionalism, which highlights the unique and sudden nature of disaster while concealing ongoing and systemic vulnerability (Luft 2009). Something obfuscated in the discourse of the triple disasters and the government's vision of smart agriculture is the longstanding disparity between rural and urban areas in Japan. Postwar economic and trade policies prioritized urbanization and industrialization at the cost of rural development. The rural population functioned as a labor reserve for the growing manufacturing industries; male economic migration left mostly women and the elderly to take care of family land (Imazato 2008). The underdevelopment and marginalization of rural areas is part of the reason that many nuclear facilities are located in such regions, due to weakened communal ties and social networks, lack of economic alternatives, and dependence on public works and subsidies (Aldrich 2010).

The place of contaminants is minimized by an affective injunction against anything that does not fit the nation's aspiration for a better collective future, and the temporality of contaminants is highly influenced by neoliberalization. The neoliberal anticipatory regime pushes the view that contaminants belong to the past, an obstacle already almost overcome and suitable to be commemorated by a nation on its way to rebirth. The government's upbeat picture of agriculture in the Tōhoku region allows only a certain place for contamination—it becomes a technical problem to be managed; in an economy that is going strong and being smart, contamination cannot cloud the vision of a bright future for the nation.

Politics of Survival

The nationalism that accelerated after the disaster sang of the excited aspirations of Japanese nationhood, but it sounded harrowing to the ears of many Japanese. Poet Hidaka Noboru (2012) shrewdly captured the post-Fukushima dynamics in a poem titled "Kimin" (Abandoned people):

> Successive governments unwilling to provide comprehensive relief
> To the Hiroshima Nagasaki A-bomb *hibakusha* [people who
>   were exposed to radiation]
> Again abandoning its people, this country
> Used to be called Zipangu
> Idolized as a place of golden rice plants waving in the wind.

The Fukushima accident feels like a reprisal of Hiroshima and Nagasaki not only because it produced hibakusha again. It is the pattern of kimin, abandoned people, that Hidaka sees in both cases. This notion, as articulated in the poem, also finds an echo in the notion of "bare life" theorized by philosopher Giorgio Agamben. He points out the normalization of a state of exception where law is suspended by the sovereign power, resulting in the condition of bare life, that is, life constantly exposed to the threat of death and unprotected by the state (Agamben 1998). The modern sovereign state seeks to maximize the population's economic productivity via control of health and wellness through various means, but ironically, the survival and well-being of individual citizens is no longer a right to be claimed vis-à-vis the government. Modern states suspend their obligations to protect citizens' basic rights, leaving many in the condition of bare life.

In her analysis of post-Chernobyl Ukraine, anthropologist Adriana Petryna observed that citizenship was redefined in a way that no longer guaranteed the protection of the life of the citizens. She says, "Protection is a legal right no longer self-evidently emanating from the state, but one whose existence is at least partially assured by citizens' everyday exercise of their democratic capacities to identify, balance, or neutralize opposing forces that give or take life" (Petryna 2002, 164). She was writing, of course, about how Ukrainians after the disaster were forced to establish a relationship with the state based on their experience of injury and damage from the nuclear accident. Governments have a stake in maintaining a healthy, productive population, but individuals are disposable, and their protection no longer an obligation.

The post-Fukushima period epitomizes the condition of bare life in many ways, and it is not surprising that kimin surfaced as a key concept in describing the situation. The accident resulted in the violation of the basic human rights of many people in the affected areas. Examples of the government's abandonment of its responsibility to protect its citizens abound. For instance, the government concealed the SPEEDI (System for Prediction of Environmental Emergency Dose Information) data that simulated the flow of radioactive materials. This resulted in the perverse evacuation of people to areas more contaminated than those they had left. The government also decided against distributing iodine pills right after the accident, which might have helped prevent thyroid cancer. The pills were, however, made available to a select few, including staff at Fukushima Medical University. They took iodine despite their official position that it was not necessary, and they did not admit that they had taken the pills until they were forced to do so by a media exposé ("Purometeus no Wana" 2013). Furthermore, the government limited thyroid screening to residents of Fukushima Prefecture despite the fact that ionizing iodine contaminated other prefectures. The government also limited which doctors people could go to for a screening, while harassing other doctors to keep them from giving second opinions ("Kujyū Hibakujirikikensa" 2014). In a paradigmatic instance of bare life, where the sovereign state's law is rendered meaningless by the hand of the state itself, the standards for the legal protection of citizens and their human rights were suspended by the government, which decided to encourage people to return to some areas despite contamination that exceeded the predisaster legal limit of 1 microsievert per year. The government was worried that evacuation based on the previous standard would be too costly.[5]

Another poet, Wakamatsu Jōtaro, wrote, "I thought I became a *nanmin* [refugee], but now I tend to think that I am a kimin" (Wakamatsu 2012,

198–99). The accident created not refugees, who were stateless people, but kimin, people whose lives were bare after they were abandoned by their own nation-state even while residing within its national borders. The government prioritized the economy over the life of its citizens, refusing to protect their health and wellness even as it simultaneously demanded that people bond in national unity to face the unprecedented national challenge.

It is in this kind of politics of bare life that I situate CRMOs. Measuring contamination to obtain safe food was an act of self-defense in a nation that was now inhabited by many kimin. Many interviewees involved in CRMOs—particularly those who had fled Fukushima and the surrounding areas—talked of their fundamental distrust of the government and compared the nuclear accident to World War II; in the words of one interviewee, "the government discarded us" (*kuni wa kokumin wo suteru*). In the mission statement of a CRMO in Fukushima, the theme of kimin and having to protect one's own life was obvious: "We who continue to live in Japan are forced to live with radiation after 3.11. . . . Each individual is required to make an effort to reduce radiation exposure. We started to test in order to gain knowledge about radiation protection, and *in order to protect ourselves, by ourselves*" (*mizukaraga mizukara wo mamorutame no sokutei*) (Nihon Iraku Iryō Shien Nettowāku 2014, 22, emphasis added). The CRMOs' mission was defined less by political ideology or electoral/legislative needs than by the livelihood needs of the moment.

The story of a man who established a CRMO in western Japan crystallizes the desperate and basic nature of the needs that motivated many CRMOs. A married man in his forties, he had an infant son only six months old when the nuclear accident happened, and his wife had just begun weaning the child and using more formula. Although the government insisted that formula was safe, and the formula company said they had stopped producing formula after the accident, contaminated formula was discovered. The government stated that the level was much lower than the standard, but these parents could not believe that it did not pose any threat to babies' health. Their concern was aggravated when their son's milk teeth came in malformed. Their pediatrician assured them that this could happen to any child, but they continued to suspect radioactive contamination. The mother's worries grew until the family was no longer living a normal life—she insisted on not using milk, eggs, domestic meat, fish, mushrooms, or anything from eastern Japan. It was increasingly hard to find anything that they could eat. The father desperately searched the web for food that was produced before the accident. Because his wife was also worried about preschool lunches, they went to talk to the school, but they were treated as if they were crazy and, in the end, told to withdraw their son from the school. This father witnessed his wife's mental state significantly deteriorating; she started saying, "It would be better to kill him [their son] now before he suffers like children in Chernobyl." They did not have enough to eat either. "I just needed something that we could eat," he said in the interview. "It's that simple." He bought a detector and started testing food for his family (and later opened it up for others who wanted to do the same).

A historian of Asia, Tessa Morris-Suzuki, observes that what she calls "informal life politics" has spread in the region, which is different from organized social mobilizations or formal democratic procedures. It refers to actions by "groups who are impelled by threats to their life, livelihood or cultural survival to engage in self-help, nongovernmental forms of actions" (Morris-Suzuki 2014a, 58). Cases like citizens' testing after the Fukushima accident might not look like a form of politics, but Morris-Suzuki argues that it ought to be considered a variant of politics that is motivated by survival needs. Survival itself has become the heart of power struggles in the contemporary world. In this context, citizen science might not become a classic social movement, and it might not look like it is worth much in lieu of policy changes or representation in legislative processes.

The CRMOs could be considered such an instance of people creating a space for survival in an effort to protect life and livelihood. This understanding could help explain why they might be precarious and rather ephemeral. As people's needs have changed, CRMO activities have also shifted to include other programs besides testing food for contamination. For instance, people near the reactors needed to know where the hot spots were so that they could ensure that their children avoided those areas. In response, some CRMOs started to conduct what might be called hot spot mapping, using a detector with geographic information system capability. Walking along the routes used daily, particularly by children (such as the roads on which they walk to school), they have created maps that are highly practical for people living in contaminated areas. Seeing that many parents in the contaminated areas wanted to evacuate but could not for various reasons, some CRMOs started coordinating short-term evacuation programs for children. Modeled after programs in Chernobyl-affected areas, children would be sent outside the affected areas so that they could enjoy outdoor activities without worrying about inhaling radiation.

People running CRMOs also face different kinds of life problems beyond food contamination, which sometimes pull them away from CRMO activities. For instance, one woman was volunteering at a CRMO in the southern region. She was an evacuee with her children, and she and her husband managed a long-distance marriage for over a year after she evacuated. They could not evacuate together because of his job and the mortgage on the house they had just bought. Even after evacuation, she was concerned about food and got involved in setting up and running the CRMO. But she was facing multiple other issues when I interviewed her in 2013. One of them was that her municipality was considering accepting a government plan to construct a new military base for the Self-Defense Force. The area had come to be of critical importance in defense against neighboring countries. She got involved in a mayoral election, which was fought between the antibase candidate and the incumbent backed by the dominant Liberal Democratic Party, who was probase. Having thought that she had brought her family to a peaceful, uncontaminated place, she now faced the increasing right-wing nationalism and militarization of the South China Sea.

Because women tend to bear the burden of caring responsibilities, their time and energy are more likely to be diverted to other pressing issues of daily livelihood. Care work—caring for children, the sick, the disabled, and the elderly—is essential for the maintenance of a family's or a community's wellness and health, and is disproportionately shouldered by women. An important finding of feminist scholarship on care is that it is often made invisible and devalued, yet it is time consuming, around the clock, hard to schedule, and physically and emotionally draining (Glenn 2000). It is not a coincidence that many CRMOs have male volunteers who are relatively young retirees. These are the people who have the most flexibility and perhaps the fewest caring responsibilities. Women, facing the different tasks of managing their own and other people's daily necessities, are often forced away from activism to address more immediate concerns. The link between the burden of care work under neoliberalism and the suppression of radical women's movements has been noticed by feminist scholars who study women's movements around the world. For instance, Rebecca Dolhinow, in her study of Mexican women in the impoverished border zone settlements called *colonias*, says, "These women are capable and resourceful, but they are also overworked and overextended. These latter two qualities, along with the neoliberal ideology at the center of colonia development, mean leaders have little extra time or energy to devote to doing political work" (2014, 175).

Care demands on women are very salient in Fukushima, especially in terms of the issue of senior care. Fukushima has experienced a significant demographic change since the nuclear accident. Depopulation had been an issue in rural areas before the accident, and the aging of the population had been more serious in the Tōhoku region than in other areas (Cabinet Office 2014b). But Fukushima's demographic problem accelerated after the accident. The prefecture lost more than 80,000 people between 2011 and 2014. The reduction of population took place in the younger groups, while the seniors (people over sixty-five years old) increased by more than 23,000 people (Yoshioka 2014). By 2014, seniors were about 27 percent of the general population in Fukushima (Fukushima Prefecture 2014), while, for instance, they were about 13 percent in the United States in 2010 (Pew Research Center 2014). Because senior care is traditionally shouldered by the women of a household (particularly the wife of the eldest son, as part of filial obligation), the accelerated aging of the region meant a dramatic increase in women's care burden.[6]

The CRMOs are endeavors by citizens who saw the bareness of the conditions of existence after the nuclear accident and tried to address it in a way that was practical for them in their daily lives. Not being able to share the excited, forward-looking attitude that rendered contaminants obsolete, these people have tried to address contaminants as a presently existing threat, rather than a risk to be mitigated and prepared for in the future. Yet the bareness of their lives simultaneously makes it difficult for them to engage with radical politics, as they are already overworked and exhausted by trying to survive in the neoliberal order.

Conclusion

This and previous chapters have examined the difficulty for CRMOs of engaging in overt forms of politics and the possibility of science replacing politics. Some readers might think that such an avoidance of politics is particularly Japanese, with Japan's uniquely strong state that effectively keeps civil society at arm's length. Historically, Japanese governments have maneuvered civil society by way of "moral suasion," even after the war, when Japanese were supposed to have transitioned from being *shinmin* (subjects) of the imperial state to being *shimin* (citizens) of a democratic country (Garon 1998, 7). Civic organizations—including many women's organizations—have long worked with, not necessarily against, the state to address various welfare, environmental, and moral issues (Garon 1998). It is also possible to attribute the lack of overt forms of politics to a unique postdisaster environment that propelled people to emphasize cooperation rather than dissent. The events of March 2011 came to be imagined as a national crisis (Dudden 2012; Sand 2012), with the emperor urging the nation's citizens to "treat each other with compassion and overcome these difficult times" ("Japan's Earthquake" 2011). The slogan Ganbarō Nippon (Don't give up, Japan) became ubiquitous, appearing on posters and billboards (Hurnung 2011). Disaster nationalism naturalized and glorified the nation as a place of *kizuna*, bonds (Dudden 2012; Sand 2012).

But people in CRMOs did not have an illusion about the state as a benevolent protector—the concept of kimin captures such awareness. Indexing the avoidance of overt politics as an instance of Japanese exceptionalism misses the chance of investigating the impacts of neoliberalization and how it demands a certain kind of attitude as the conduct of good citizenship. Neoliberal citizen-subjects are to resourcefully protect themselves to be aspiring economic agents even in the shadow of progressively weakened social protection, income stratification, and environmental hazards. What was striking about the Fukushima case was how they claimed the status of shimin as a counterpoint to the discredited experts and technocrats, and yet being shimin-as-neoliberal-citizens often paralyzed their ability to become politically active.

But even when politics with a capital P might be difficult, that does not mean that there is no politics. James C. Scott's (1990, 2008) concepts of "infrapolitics" and "hidden resistance" describe acts of resistance that, while far from revolution and uprising, are often more effective in gaining some social and economic benefits for the marginalized. Other theorists have proposed similar ideas, pointing out subversive actions by regular people that take place under the radar of mainstream politics (Bayat 2013; Kerkvliet 1990).

Concepts such as informal life politics (Morris-Suzuki 2014a) and "imperceptible politics" (Papadopoulos, Stephenson, and Tsianos 2008) similarly point out that the linkage between something outside of the classic conceptualization of social movements is taking place. Imperceptible politics, according to Papadopoulos and his colleagues, refers to "social change in experiences that point towards an exit from a given organisation of social life without ever intending to create an event . . . these moments where people subvert their existing situations without naming their practice" (xiii).

In the Japanese studies literature, too, anthropologist Anne Allison has discussed a kind of mobilization that differs from traditional social movements, a "biopolitics of life from below" (2012, 346). In what she calls "precarious Japan," where many youths are without the prospect of decent employment, and many seniors have to address their medical and daily needs on their own as the social protection afforded by the government has shrunk, traditional social movements have been severely handicapped in their ability to address people's practical life needs. Would resistance to the regime of power in such cases be limited to "simply the resistance against dying; the will to keep living," as Allison hypothetically asked? Rather, she sees resistance in "extra-economic networks of survival" in such places as a café for *hikikomori* (people who withdraw from society) and poetry events for suicide seekers. These people are connecting to create a space for survival.

That CRMOs are such a form of survival politics was clear, for instance, in my interview with Tomita Tokiko. I was taken by surprise when she suddenly started talking about *nenkin*—a slime mold. I was asking her about her CRMO and its challenges and, in a seeming detour, she said, "Do you know about nenkin? Those in the *nattō* [fermented beans]? I saw this on television but they are very cool. . . . When the environment is harsh, like a long period of no rain, they gather and make a colony to weather it. When it rains, they start telling each other and start moving toward the better conditions." She continued, "We need to be like nenkin. Right now it is so hard, we are so exhausted, so we might need to just weather it." She hunched her body to demonstrate as she went on, "We need to save our mental and physical strength. And the nenkin don't have any leaders . . . but if we can nurture our sensor that tells us when to move, then we can move in the right direction together. And you know, they don't have a leader, but they also don't leave out anyone. . . . They move everyone."

A CRMO was like nenkin to her, a move to survive in harsh conditions. She envisioned herself as part of the slime mold colony, which acted to preserve itself without much hierarchical structure, leadership, or even a clear sense of direction. The CRMO was a place to "nurture our sensor" so as to know how to move to protect one's life.

Tomita-san operates a natural food restaurant in Fukushima, which also houses a CRMO. She has had substantial experience in what we might see as social movement activism. In the 1990s, she established an NGO that concentrated on sustainable living and farming. After the nuclear accident, she got involved in various policy issues, and took part in petitions, rallies, demonstrations, and direct negotiations with government agencies. I met her in 2013 and 2014, and it was clear that as the years passed following the accident, her frustration was growing. After three years and practically no change in the government's pronuclear policy, she said she felt "exhausted and beaten" (*kutakuta, boroboro*).

She was also seeing the coming of a health crisis in her area, which was in Fukushima Prefecture and had a relatively high radiation level at over 0.4 microsieverts per hour in March 2011 and 0.1–0.3 microsieverts per hour in March 2014 (while 0.04–0.06 was the preaccident level). As for many other parents in Fukushima, radiation-induced thyroid cancer had become a real concern for her. One of her children had been diagnosed A2 in a thyroid ultrasound diagnostic test, which meant that some nodules and cysts had been identified. While the government and experts said that there was no need to be concerned by an A2 diagnosis (Fukushima Prefecture and Fukushima Medical University 2013), she was still worried. She also talked about the need to care for the elderly. She said, "I am thinking of starting a worker cooperative for taking care of the elderly," as she saw that others in the community were also increasingly facing elder care needs since so many more younger people than older ones had evacuated. With layers of caring responsibilities—in her case, child care, sick care, and elder care—Tomita-san epitomized the situation of many women who were struggling to respond to one care need after another.

With their lack of formal organizing and their tenuous financial bases, CRMOs seem rather ephemeral. In addition, many women involved in

CRMOs, like Tomita-san, face constantly changing life needs in their families and communities. While we might consider CRMOs an example of underresourced NGOs, perhaps sustaining an organizational basis is beside the point.

But the situation raises many questions that remain unanswered. Why were people forced to engage in this type of politics as abandoned people? The precariousness of CRMOs also suggests that the measurement data they have provided and the informal know-how and practical tips on operating detectors might not be preserved in the long run. If the CRMOs disappear, the response in the case of another Fukushima will not be as prompt as it could be if they survive. Another Chernobyl will not happen, the nuclear establishment declared after 1986. Given the aging of nuclear reactors, particularly in a nation prone to earthquakes, CRMOs might, unfortunately, prove indispensable to ensuring food safety in the future as well. But the dominant view emphasizes smart preparedness to deal with future contamination, not the prevention of similar tragedies. Furthermore, it obfuscates the struggles of women with contaminants here and now.

In this constraining climate of neoliberal dispossession, citizen science can be a means for self-protection as well as for speaking to power. Citizen science might enable the marginalized to increase their legitimacy in partaking in scientized talks and policy decisions and in providing the data that would cajole some favorable responses from authority. Yet citizen scientists, particularly women, have to juggle diverse livelihood needs that are also accelerated due to contamination, neoliberal cuts in social services, and increasing economic stratification and competition. Choreography of citizen science vacillates among different meanings, defying simple understanding of it as either heroic resistance or conformist self-help.

CONCLUSION

Monks in black robes swinging brooms, young women in kimonos, the smiling station master of Fukushima Station: all are dancing to Pharrell Williams's global blockbuster song, "Happy," in a video titled "Fukushima Happy" that became a social media hit in Japan in 2014. Kumasaka Hitomi, who made the video, said that she wanted to show that "although the typical image of Fukushima is a dark city where all the residents are walking around with their faces covered by masks, most people are living a regular, happy life." Originally from Fukushima, she was "angered by *Oishinbo*" (the comic discussed in chapter 1) and wanted to combat fūhyōhigai. The message of her video was that "there might be unhappy people, but there do exist many happy people in Fukushima. And here in Fukushima too, there is a bright future as well" (Kumasaka 2014). Despite contamination and depopulation, Fukushima "will be just fine," as the lyrics go, and chooses to be "happy."

This book has explored how citizen science figures in the prevailing policing and avoidance of overt forms of politics where ordinary citizens struggle to become both citizen scientists and political citizens. Neoliberalism's impact is critical; its framing of politics as negative is coupled with its injunction to maximize emotional potential and to be forward looking. Like the dancing people in "Fukushima Happy," neoliberal citizens are to be happy; they are to choose to be happy—perhaps despite the lack of meaningful choices. The dictum to be happy makes it difficult to be outraged about injustices and inequality, particularly for women, who are even more subject to cultural mandates to be obedient and nice. The book has documented how the ideal neoliberal citizen as a self-responsible, resourceful, and forward-looking actor is performed through science.

I have also pointed to complex manifestations of the agency of citizens, and of women in particular. Various theorists have noted that a lack of revolution and large demonstrations does not necessarily mean that no civic actions are taking place, as James Scott's concepts of "infrapolitics" (1990) and "hidden resistance" (2008), Asef Bayat's "social nonmovements" (2013, 4), and Tessa Morris-Suzuki's "informal life politics" (2014a) help make evident. These scholars have pointed out that subaltern people engage in actions that might not look like much but still chip away at the space occupied by authorities, and have the potential to collectively gain concessions and recognition from the elites.

The book's contribution to this literature is to draw on science and technology studies and think about the role of citizen science in invisible politics. The book has pointed out how citizen science actions could be a way to improve people's lot without seeming overtly political. But not all citizen science is the same. Citizen science can be about doing technical data gathering, but it can also be a practice for social change. In the cases examined in this book, the degree of politicization varied among the post-Fukushima citizen scientists. Many CRMOs tried hard to strike a balance between politics and science, weighing efficacy, legitimacy, and practical needs differently at different times.

This finding that even seemingly similar citizen scientists (say, CRMOs) have different degrees of politicization calls for researchers to give their attention to the different activities of citizen scientists rather than simply indexing all citizen science as inherently civic-minded political engagement.[1] While the science and technology studies literature has tended to focus on citizen science's scientific contribution, the prevailing scientism makes it important that citizen science bring justice concerns back into the conversation. We can think of citizen science's political contribution in terms of two types of justice: epistemic and procedural. Epistemic justice is about how subaltern groups ought not to be denied the possibility of being the knowers and the knowledge producers. Procedural justice relates to how citizens ought to participate in making decisions that will affect their lives (Fricker 2007).

This book has shown how citizen science can both enable and constrain these two justices. In relation to epistemic justice, on the one hand, citizen science can counter knowledge gaps and "undone science"

(Frickel et al. 2010; Hess 2009), producing knowledge that matters and is meaningful to regular citizens. For instance, CRMOs test food from home gardens that the government screening system does not screen, and also give data to those citizens who want to know about even below-standard levels of contamination. But at the same time, citizen science could accelerate scientization if its problematization remains within the bounds of technical questions at the cost of social justice and distributive questions.

In relation to procedural justice, citizen science can help regular people gain some legitimacy to take part in policy discussions. But at the same time, citizen science can also help to accelerate the reductionist construction of problems as technoscientific, marginalizing those who do not wish to discuss the issue as strictly scientific or who are seen as less qualified to speak in such terms. The book has shown, for instance, how women in the safe school lunch groups were particularly pressured to take up science to gain legitimacy to speak on what was considered a technical-scientific problem of contamination, but even when they did so, they were often shut out from decision-making processes.

I point to the concept of justice (both epistemic and procedural) as an important counterpoint to the idea of happiness. The neoliberal and postfeminist injunction to have it all, including happiness, makes anger and outrage about injustices unfashionable. When contamination escapes human senses and its impacts are not acute, choosing to be happy is seductive or necessary if there is no other option but to live with it. Bringing justice concerns back into scientized conversation—this is the role that the book calls on citizen scientists to claim.

This book has examined how ordinary citizens, particularly many laywomen, acted as citizen scientists to detect possible contamination in food after the Fukushima nuclear accident. They went against the official position that held food safety to be largely ensured, government screening to be thorough, and regulatory standards to be rigorous enough. They opened up testing services for fellow citizens and fostered safe spaces for citizens to share information and concerns. Unlike many studies on citizen science, the story in this book is not a simple contestation of science and technocracy by laypeople. Citizen scientists in neoliberal and postfeminist regimes face great challenges in scientization and depoliticization. Citizen science can be a way to perform the requirements of citizens in such regimes, but it can also be a way to somehow try to subvert them. The intersections of contamination and social inequality and the increasing difficulties of democratic participation in science-based policy making that this book has described crystallize the need for citizen science that pushes for not only a happier but also a more just society.

NOTES

Introduction

1. The Geiger counter, which measures radiation in the air, cannot measure small amounts of radioactive materials in food. Measurement of gamma rays in food requires special detectors that are able to block background radiation so as to measure only what is in the food. What was usually used by citizen radiation-measuring stations is called a scintillation spectrometer.

2. "Citizen science" refers to the involvement of laypeople in creating knowledge that is scientifically relevant. The term is usually credited to a British social scientist, Alan Irwin. In his 1995 book, *Citizen Science*, he describes how environmental contamination was forcing laypeople to learn about scientific issues and how in turn they came to contribute to science itself. A related concept is "popular epidemiology," which, according to Phil Brown (1993), refers to laypeople detecting and challenging environmental hazards.

3. The website for the Ministry of Health, Labor, and Welfare maintains a database of food radiation levels tested by the government every month at http://www .mhlw.go.jp/.

4. The actual level of exposure from food (excluding external radiation) by the average Japanese person after the Fukushima accident was estimated to be somewhere between 0.003 to 0.023 mSv (Government of Japan 2012).

5. These data are from the Japanese Ministry of Agriculture, Forestry and Fisheries (2014) and Fisheries Agency (2014); http://www.jfa.maff.go.jp/j/housyanou /pdf/1410_kousin.pdf.

6. Tessa Morris-Suzuki (2014a) draws on Rancière's notion of politics to argue the need for broadening the conceptualization of politics. This issue is expanded more in chapter 4.

7. For Rancière, politics is always disruptive of the police order. Politics, according to him, is about declassification, where people abandon an already-given

identity, and about dissensus, which disrupts an existing social order. As he says, "political action . . . is always a matter of knowing who is qualified to say what a particular place is and what is done to it" (Rancière 2003, 201).

8. Scholars have also found that the historical formation of the modern state was intricately linked to modern technoscience, through which the state rendered people, land, and other materials governable and symbolic of state power (Mukerji 1994, 2002, 2009).

9. In fact, Western societies have long seen science as an ideal civic activity. Various philosophers of science have argued that science and democracy are highly compatible. Robert Merton (1973), for instance, considered four values of science— communality, universalism, disinterestedness, and organized skepticism—to be the basis of democratic society. Despite science's track record of objectification and exploitation of human subjects, heterosexism, and patriarchal attitudes (Harding 1991), the argument that science embodies prototypical civic virtues is still made today (Koertge 2005).

10. "Ecological modernization" refers to the idea that environmental protection is compatible with economic development in a win-win situation. Scientific and technical expertise play a key role in it (Mol 2003). It has been criticized, for instance from ecofeminist perspectives, as putting too much emphasis on technical and regulatory solutions (Bäckstrand 2004).

11. Minamata (mercury poisoning) was caused by toxic waste from chemical plants operated by the Chisso Corporation in Kumamoto Prefecture. The first human victim was recorded in 1953, and later thousands of people claimed they had the disease. After a long legal battle, Chisso finally agreed to pay compensation to the victims (George 2001). Itai-itai byo (cadmium poisoning) was caused by the Mitsui Metal-Mining Company's mining plant in Toyama Prefecture, first reported in 1955. Yokkaichi asthma was related to an industrial complex built in the 1950s in Mie Prefecture. A small group of victims filed suit against several of the plants and were finally recognized as victims (Wilkening 2004). Historian B. Walker says that in these cases, "it is fair to say that the courts favored the victims" (2009, 218).

12. Another example of the ecological modernization view is Wilkening's assessment drawn from the analysis of acid rain policies in Japan. He wrote, "Even though direct channels for citizen input into policymaking are essentially nonexistent, public opinion expressed via the mass media (the major vehicle for citizen input) nonetheless provides a constant reminder to the central government that its citizens, who often see the acid deposition problem through a cultural lens, want clean rain and green forests. This, in turn, bolsters bureaucrats' resolve to tackle the problem. If bureaucrats waiver, there are tens of thousands who will notice" (Wilkening 2004, 210).

13. There were many accidents at Japanese nuclear power plants before the Fukushima accident, including an explosion at the Tokaimura power plant in 1999, which killed several workers.

1. "Moms with Radiation Brain"

1. Note that at this point, the government was still using the provisionary regulatory values, which were more lax than standards adopted later and in effect today.

2. The Ministry of Health issued a notice (No. 0317 Article 3 of the Department of Food Safety), saying, "'Indexes Relating to Limits on Food and Drink Ingestion' by the Nuclear Safety Commission shall be adopted for the time being as provisional regulation values, and foods which exceed these levels shall be deemed to be regulated by Article 6, Item 2 of the Food Sanitation Act" (Ministry of Health, Labor, and Welfare 2011).

3. In contrast, Ukraine, for instance, has stricter standards for staples such as potatoes at 70 Bq/kg and bread at 20 Bq/kg for cesium (Foodwatch 2011).

4. See Kimura (2013b) on the social contestation of the setting of the new standards.

5. Even in 2014, three years after the accident, a survey by the Fukushima Chamber of Commerce of consumers in the Tokyo metropolitan area found that about 30 percent of the respondents did not buy Fukushima food ("Fukushimakensan-hinkawanai 30%" 2014).

6. According to a government survey, the population of Fukushima Prefecture decreased by 1.93 percent from October 2010 to October 2011 (Ministry of Internal Affairs and Communications 2012). Between 2011 and 2014, the population in Fukushima decreased by 4 percent, a loss of about 80,000 people (Yoshioka 2014).

7. Other groups argued that it was a suppression of freedom of expression as well as denial of actual experiences of nasal bleeding and other health impacts that might not have been validated by official science but were nonetheless true in the eyes of those who experienced them ("*Oishinbo* Hyōgen Ni Zannen; Kankyōshō Seimukan" 2014).

8. The reasons respondents gave for their concern included the unprecedented nature of the accident, the lack of consensus among scientists, and the lack of information disclosure by the government. Gendered concern in regard to food safety can also be seen in the case of genetically modified organisms (GMOs). On average, men have more positive attitudes toward GMOs than women (Tanaka 2007).

9. This gendered pattern of radiation concern could be interpreted in various ways. Some experts—including scientists and regulatory agencies in fields related to nuclear energy—tend to see women's concerns about contamination as a sign of women's lack of knowledge and scientific literacy. In popular discourse, on the other hand, women are often considered to be especially sensitive to contamination issues because of an innate connection or closeness to nature—a view perhaps most clearly captured by ecofeminist arguments that women's reproductive function puts them in better sync with nature's rhythms. Many feminist theorists have argued that neither of these views of women captures the nuances of women's relationship to contamination, instead positing that it is women's social positions—as

mothers, wives, and caregivers—that make them feel the day-to-day impacts of toxic contamination more intensely than men (Mollett and Faria 2013). Geographer Joni Seager wrote, "Because women, worldwide, still have primary responsibility for feeding, housing, and childcare, they are often the first to notice when the water smells peculiar, when the laundry gets dingier with each wash, when children develop mysterious ailments—or they are the first to worry that these assaults on family safety and health are imminent. This may appear to be a humble entry point for environmental awareness, but in fact it has catalyzed a powerful environmental challenge at the grassroots. Moreover, environmental degradation is typically mundane: it occurs in small measures, drop by drop, well by well, tree by tree" (1996, 280).

10. In July 2014, the operator of the Fukushima Daiichi nuclear reactors, TEPCO, admitted that the decontamination work at the troubled plant probably resulted in the spread of cesium. This was many months after farmers reported unusually high levels of cesium in rice that could not be explained based on already deposited cesium ("Minami-Soma Lambastes Government" 2014; Terashima 2014).

11. Some even argued that the hysterical mothers were damaging not only food producers but their own children. Journalist Ishii Takaaki, for instance, wrote about the "radiation panic" of mothers, saying, "I particularly want to appeal to mothers. Mothers have the biggest impact on children under ten years old. You should not put them in a situation where they feel hatred against the government and the corporations. The fear and anger of mothers can infect children. . . . I consider concerns after the Fukushima accident unwise. Most probably there will be no damage to health, and the current confusion in society and individual lives is out of proportion" (Ishii 2012).

12. Since 2003, atomic bomb victims have filed close to twenty lawsuits against the government arguing that its certification system was flawed and its definition of exposure too narrow. Most of the lawsuits have been decided in favor of the victims. It is noteworthy that some of the court decisions pointed to the problem of lack of research on internal radiation by ABCC/RERF, despite the fact that the victim data became the basis for international standard setting (see, for instance, Osaka High Court 2008).

13. In another document, RERF similarly admitted its lack of knowledge on internal radiation: "It is not an exaggeration to conclude that the estimation of amounts of inhalation of radioactive substances in the air and of intake from food and drink (internal exposure dose) is nearly impossible" (Radiation Effects Research Foundation 2012, 2).

14. Many see the ICRP as part of the international nuclear establishment whose interest has historically been closely aligned with the nuclear industry. Historian Nakagawa Yasuo, for instance, chronicled the development of nuclear-related institutions and observed that the "ICRP is an international committee that has brought economic and political benefits to the nuclear industry and the elites at the cost of radiation to regular citizens" (Nakagawa 1991, 296). He pointed out that the ICRP

was established under the strong influence of the US National Council on Radiation Protection, whose members included Robert S. Stone and Stafford L. Warren of the Manhattan Project. It worked closely with the United States to minimize the issue of health damage from radiation, which threatened to sway public opinion against the US atmospheric nuclear bomb testing program.

15. For a point-by-point criticism of the UNSCEAR report, see Physicians for Social Responsibility et al. (2013).

16. The Food Safety Commission's Kubo Junichi also admitted an absence of data on food-based internal radiation and its health effects. At a conference in 2012, he said, "Unfortunately (when considering the new standards), it would have been good to base them on data on food-based internal radiation, but such data were almost nonexistent" (Kubo 2012, 7).

17. At least fourteen Aeon stores were found to have sold about 420 kg of the cesium-contaminated beef. Aeon tested agricultural produce from its own seven farms, with one test per week on samples. For its private-brand products, it asked contract farmers to test samples once before shipment. In September 2011, it started to test samples of rice from each silo. For fish, Aeon measured radiation levels on a sample of select varieties (salmon, mackerel, bonito, and saury) once a week (Kanda, Nagai, and Shinohara 2011).

18. Itō-Yōkadō started testing all beef in August 2011 after it was found to have sold 2,651 kg of contaminated beef at ninety-four stores ("Itō-Yōkadō Sold Beef" 2011).

19. This network was created by a female activist, Haruka Fujii, from a nonprofit organization called the Network to Protect Children from Radiation, and involved largely small and independent cafés and restaurants. The criteria they set for the members were that the restaurant needed either to use produce from unaffected areas, to adopt stricter standards than the government standards, or to test ingredients. They also had to disclose detailed information on their radiation strategy.

2. Engineering Citizens

1. Nelson wrote about a public relations campaign by the US nuclear industry in the 1980s: "Not surprisingly, the industry is directing its message to liberal feminism. Liberal feminists' desire to participate fully and assertively in a reformed liberal capitalism is being addressed by industry propagandists who assert that nuclear and a high-growth economy will provide for a reversal of discrimination, sustain women's already hard-won gains, and guarantee the evolution of equality" (1984, 299–300).

2. Similarly, legal scholar Tokuda Hiroto summarized the attitude toward risk communication in the Food Safety Basic Law by saying, "Citizens do not understand that there is zero risk and we need to make them understand the notion of risk analysis," which he criticizes as a betrayal of the original intent of the law (Tokuda 2003, 2).

3. The desire to enlist laypeople into risk communication existed before the Fukushima nuclear accident. For instance, in 2006, the government issued the Third Basic Plan for Science and Technology, which emphasized the need for risk communication on technoscientific issues in general. This plan called for "risk communicators" who would help form social consensus on controversial technoscientific issues (Yagi 2007).

4. To be more precise, the training consists of an orientation by Consumer Affairs Agency staff (twenty minutes), a lecture on basic knowledge of radiation (sixty–ninety minutes), a lecture about food and radiation by agency staff, the showing of the DVD "Food and Radiation Q and A," and a lecture on public speaking on the first day. The second day includes a follow-up session facilitated by agency staff and a lecture on radiation, plus a question and answer session. Many participants are recruited from the Japan Dietetic Association, Nippon Association of Consumer Specialists, and Japanese Association of Food Science and Risk Analysis, but there are also participants who are not from these organizations.

5. The other organization is the Japan Science Foundation, established in the 1960s with the objective of promoting science and technology education and under the jurisdiction of the Ministry of Education and the Ministry of Economy, Trade, and Industry.

6. Their use of lay citizens is not unusual, and perhaps is increasingly common. The newspaper *Tokyo Shinbun* reported on "citizen groups" hired by local municipal governments in Fukushima Prefecture to give more than eighty lectures on radiation dangers. But the groups were decidedly pronuclear, and one of their spokespeople was quoted as saying, "the scale of explosion at Fukushima was very different from Chernobyl. So there is nothing to worry about" (Sakakibara 2014).

7. These numbers are for 2014, and it is estimated that the figure will increase.

8. They are held in conjunction with the Japanese nuclear lobbying group, Radiation Safety Forum Japan, the Fukushima prefectural government, and Fukushima Medical University. Financial support comes from the French Institute of Radiation Protection and Nuclear Safety, Norwegian Radiation Protection Authority, and the Nuclear Energy Agency's Committee on Radiation Protection and Public Health for the Organisation for Economic Co-operation and Development (Lochard 2012).

9. For instance, ICRP proclaims that it "emphasises the effectiveness of directly involving the affected population and local professionals in the management of the situation, and the responsibility of authorities at both national and local levels to create the conditions and provide the means favouring the involvement and empowerment of the population" (Lochard et al. 2009, 1).

10. For instance, Ishibashi Suomi, now a board member of WiN, recounted her struggle in the mostly male nuclear field: "There were no female seniors in the nuclear department. I lost hope. I was not the type to hate my job or get discouraged, but I was plagued with hard-to-articulate worries about my future." That was when she encountered WiN: "I am so blessed to have met role models through WiN whom I

would not have met within my company. . . . Women that I met at international WiN conferences are attractive, such as the head of a nuclear power plant who brought her child to the conference (French) and a head of PR who told me that she was working the day before she gave birth to her child" (Ishibashi 2007, 29).

11. For instance, she said, "Here I think women have great duty to fulfill because they for themselves argue emotionally. Moreover motherhood brings ethical values much closer to them" (Aegerter 1989, 2).

12. The group name in English is their translation. The group's Japanese name is Nihon no asu wo kangaeru joshigakusei fōramu.

13. Tellingly, the forum's leader saw another role model in Margaret Thatcher. In the forum's mission statement, she wrote, "Margaret Thatcher AKA Iron Woman, is known as a great prime minister who aggressively pursued reform toward smaller government. . . . What is clear is that however much she was opposed and criticized, she kept her strong will. She emotionally moves us, and her death became a global headline even 23 years after she stepped down from the prime ministerial position, because she lived her life earnestly and with passion. We want to be like her, who worked hard and kept her passion despite being vilified."

3. School Lunches

1. For instance, Chiba City officially posted its policy of allowing students to bring their own lunches and drinks if the students did not want to participate in the school lunch program. In Tokyo, thirty-two municipal governments formally allowed school lunch exemptions as official policy while the other sixteen did not ("Onajikondatede Bentō" 2012).

2. There have been controversies around whether the failure of some parents to pay the school lunch fees is due to true economic hardship or not. Some newspaper articles have tended to frame it as analogous to welfare cheating, which echoes the conservative inclination to demonize the poor for abusing social services. I could not find data to convincingly show that the failure to pay was not due to poverty. Furthermore, public assistance to the poor has been declining over the past decades, given the neoliberal restructuring of the welfare system in Japan as well.

3. These statistics are for schools that provide what is called complete school lunch, a meal consisting of rice or bread, a main dish, and milk. Other schools provide supplementary foods or milk only.

4. Similarly, when mandarin oranges were found to be contaminated and were removed from school lunches in Yokohama City and Kamakura, the producer associations lobbied fiercely against such actions, which they deemed unnecessary because the contamination did not exceed the government standard. In Odawara City, mandarin orange growers lobbied the legislature to issue a declaration that asked municipalities not to avoid their product, as the contamination was well below the standard (Odawara City Council 2012). And in Tochigi Prefecture, beef

producers also lobbied the municipal government to serve their product in school lunches.

5. The testing was effective in preventing the inclusion of contaminated food. For instance, in fiscal year 2011, eleven samples contained cesium, such as dried shiitake mushrooms, which had over 350 Bq/kg. Although this was lower than the government standard, the city government decided not to include the mushrooms in the following day's lunch (Yoshizawa 2011).

6. The mass media have also reported similar cases of criticism of the safe school lunch movement. For instance, a viewer commenting on a national television program on the topic wrote, "Families who make children eat homemade lunch instead of school lunch are arrogant, selfishly concerned only about their own children. Not buying Tōhoku produce is also a good example of fūhyōhigai, because it is said to be safe" ("Shutoken Supesharu" 2011). Many school authorities chided parents who raised concerns about school lunches. The newspaper *Mainichi Shinbun* reported that the mother of an elementary school child in Fukushima who decided to prepare homemade lunches was phoned by the principal, who told her, "School lunch is part of education. It is important to share the same meal." A report in November 2011 by the nonprofit organization Human Rights Now found many schools did not allow homemade lunches to be brought in, and the majority of parents did not dare to ask for such an option. A mother of three was quoted as saying, "I am afraid that people would see me as a 'monster parent.' There are fewer people who will speak up—because the people who would speak up have already evacuated" (Human Rights Now 2011b, 15). Concerned parents have been criticized not only by the schools but by relatives and friends. Bullying is a significant concern. Students are reported to have been bullied as being *hikenmin* (antiprefecture) for not drinking milk at school ("Twenty-Five out of Forty-Three Fukushima Vegetables" 2011). Mothers sometimes have to fight within their own households to voice their concerns. The comments of a mother of two children in Fukushima point to how tension can emerge between wife and husband: "My husband says that my kids should not do differently when it is the government's decision to provide local milk and rice. I am opposed, but I cannot evacuate or get a divorce to refuse him" (Human Rights Now 2011b, 15). Similar tensions between mothers and fathers were also reported by Rika Morioka (2014).

7. The whole-meal sample method means that testing is done after the fact, so it is mainly for research and tracking purposes, and does not reflect mothers' wishes to prevent the intake of contaminated food by their children (Makishita 2013, 48–49).

8. Note that this cutoff point is already much lower than the national standard. The official national standard for regular food has been 100 Bq/kg since April 2012.

9. Similarly, Chiba City tested mushrooms at 8.3 Bq/kg but went ahead and used them in school lunches (Makishita 2013, 53). The same thing happened in Kawasaki City ("Kodomotachino" 2012).

10. In Fukushima, forty-five municipalities (villages and cities) adopted stricter standards than the national government's recommendation of 40 Bq/kg (My Town Fukushima 2012). Cities such as Sapporo in Hokkaido and Koganei in Tokyo also declared that if a food contained more than a specific MDC, they would not use it in school lunches. Koganei's MDC was 10 Bq/kg, and Sapporo's 4 Bq/kg.

11. For instance, a group in Tokyo lobbied the municipal government to measure strontium. The government finally agreed in 2014. The testing will take place only once a year, but it became famous as it was the first instance of such a commitment (Association to Protect Children in Shinagawa 2014).

12. The session ("Kyūshokuniyoru" 2014) can be viewed on this website: http://www.hide-fujino.com/blog/2014/01/30/17662.

13. This quotation is taken from a video recording of the meeting with the mayor that is available online ("Shichōni Kōkaishitumonjō" 2012).

14. On the one hand, some scholars have found joshi to be a term that emphasizes comradeship and bonds among women, and it is often chosen by women themselves to avoid gender stereotypes. Sociologist Kawahara Kazue argues that joshi "seem to be freed from 'stereotypical values' . . . by redefining themselves and establishing homosocial networks" (Kawahara 2012, 27). But others have found that the joshi image operates within gender stereotypes that see the ultimate value of women in outward appearance and heterosexual marriage (Minashita 2013).

15. The group participated in a symposium titled "Let's Get Rid of Nuclear Reactors from Fukushima" in 2013. On the other hand, the group was featured on the Tōhoku Electricity Power Company (2014) website under the title "Transforming the World by Kawaii [cuteness]: Only Young Women Can Do It." While this company is not the same as TEPCO, it operates nuclear power plants and is in close alliance with TEPCO.

16. This group is also emblematic of activist joshi's appeal to cuteness and a self-portrayal that is conscious of a heterosexual gaze. Their website features photos of the members, who are all young women, with personal profiles including blood type, hobby, and the type of men that they are attracted to, evoking something like a dating website.

17. Tellingly, Peach Heart's leader once explained that "not trying so hard" (muri sezu) was a key phrase defining their programs, reflecting the aversion to the politically incorrect (see Morioka 2014) emotions of anger and outrage. She said that perhaps their joshi activities might seem lukewarm (nurui) to activists who are "angry and hot" but that they "want to convey [their opinions] in a relaxed manner [yuruku]," not with "something like anger or resentment about Fukushima" ("Dentōkōgei Ni 'Kawaii'" 2014).

18. The newspaper Asahi Shinbun reported in July 2011 that several municipalities were conducting tests, including Yokohama City, Kawasaki City, Maebashi City, Musashino City, Shibuya and Setagaya wards in Tokyo, and Kyoto City ("Kyūshokuno Shokuzai" 2011). In November 2011, Fukushima City started a similar

measurement program, followed by other municipalities in Fukushima Prefecture ("Kyūshokuni Hōshanōkijyun" 2011).

19. The program covered seventeen prefectures and subsidized the purchase of five detectors per prefecture specifically for the purpose of testing school lunches.

20. Although it was a step in the right direction, the national government's support for local testing was not sufficient. The subsidy was only for detectors and did not include the cost of extra meals to be used as samples for testing. The cost of personnel who would perform the tests was not included. Given the broad budget constraints that the school lunch programs face, some observers worried that many municipalities might be forced to cut back on testing soon (Makishita 2013). In 2013, the program was already cut back to nine prefectures (Aomori, Iwate, Miyagi, Fukushima, Ibaraki, Tochigi, Chiba, Niigata, and Nagano) (Shimizu 2013).

21. The groups have tried to protest the use of local rice by collecting signatures and petitioning governments. For instance, the group in Fukushima City started a signature drive and submitted a petition to the city government, but it did not get the support of the majority of the city council members. Another group in Iwaki City also submitted a petition to the mayor, arguing for reconsideration of the local rice use policy.

4. Citizen Radiation-Measuring Organizations

1. For instance, studies of social movements such as LGBT movements in the United States have pointed out how they evolved to suppress dissent, radicalism, and (in a contradictory fashion) diversity (Duggan 2012; Ghaziani 2008).

2. Some websites listed more than seventy-four CRMOs, but some of them could not be reached and hence were deemed inactive; they were not included in the total number.

3. It was possible that the risk of contamination was higher in the samples brought to CRMOs as some were foods from home gardens and from foraging not screened by the government testing procedures.

4. On the political right, the nuclear disaster could be seen as contaminating the sacred national land. The *netto uyoku* (Internet right wing) mobilized discourses of "protecting our mountains and rivers," which in the end might not be "that different from the most leftist groups" (Suga 2012, 37).

5. The New Left's involvement in antinuclear issues was not new. Although it might seem surprising from the Japan Communist Party's antinuclear platform after the Fukushima disaster, the socialist and communist parties in Japan for some time took the position of approving the "peaceful use of nuclear power," which was considered qualitatively different from nuclear weapons and promising as part of an anti-US hegemony strategy. In contrast, the New Left prided itself on taking the antinuclear position. Historian Suga Hidemi explains that, for instance, in 1962,

Nemoto Jin, chairperson of a New Left faction, Zengakuren (All-Japan Federation of Students' Self-Governing Associations), protested in Red Square in Moscow against the Soviet Union's nuclear tests. But as they focused on various other issues in the 1970s, nuclear issues were given less priority (Suga 2012, 109). The nuclear disaster made it once again one of their central missions.

6. A National Public Security Intelligence Agency report mentioned MDS in the context of anti–Iraq War protests. The report says that the MDS initiative, the "nondefended localities movement," was at its height in 2005–6 and was successful in several municipalities (Public Security Intelligence Agency 2006). However, it should also be noted that the Agency also includes in the report the activities by the Japan Communist Party.

7. Similarly, Ando Takemasa, a sociologist at Musashi University, wrote in his book, *Japan's New Left Movements*, about how the New Left was stigmatized as violent and extreme, and many local movements tried to shun it (Ando 2014, 165).

8. At another CRMO, the volunteer laywomen became quite astute readers of data on food contamination. For example, in April 2013, Shinano City in Nagano Prefecture published data on ingredients for school lunches. For April 5, it showed that cabbage from Aichi Prefecture contained 7.86 ± 6.64 Bq/kg. Again on April 10, it showed 10.25 ± 8.71. When the volunteer saw the data, she thought it was strange. In the interview, she said, "this cannot be true, I thought. Ten Bq/kg from cabbage from this area was just too high to be true. I had come to know the pattern of what kind of things can be contaminated, and this was so unusual that I suspected an error." To find out, her CRMO obtained cabbages from the same area in Aichi, and found that they were not contaminated (below nondetectable level). The city later admitted the measurement error (Nagoya Seikatsu Kurabu n.d.).

9. This measurement was made with a germanium detector.

10. For instance, important debates have taken place on how to include nonhumans in the conception of politics. Following the path expanded by actor-network theory that insists upon the inclusion of nonhumans in thinking about sociotechnical dynamics, the notion of the politics of ontology includes how the existence of stuff, including nonhuman stuff, becomes real. A concept proposed by Papadopoulos (2011), "constituent politics," for instance, indicates an interest in understanding the process in which an entity becomes an entity as constituting politics, rather than a mere precondition for it. As he defines it, constituent politics is an "attempt to create material alliances between particular groups of people and particular non-human others in order to confront injustice and to make new conditions that ultimately challenge how a certain region of objectivity works. . . . Constituent politics are neither acts of opposition nor of renegotiation of the architectures of power; rather constituent politics attempt to think through and *literally* make alternative forms of sociability and materiality" (194, emphasis in original). Testing can result in such forms of politics, enacting a certain reality and shifting a political conversation.

11. Also see the special issue on the topic in the journal *Social Studies of Science* (Woolgar and Lezaun 2013a).

5. The Temporality of Contaminants

1. "Vegetables" excludes bamboo shoots, wild herbs, mushrooms, beans, and rice. Mushrooms and wild herbs tend to have higher odds of contamination. For instance, 194 out of 7,581 samples in the category of wild herbs and mushrooms exceeded 100 Bq/kg in 2013 (Ministry of Agriculture, Forestry and Fisheries 2014).

2. For instance, TEPCO admitted in 2002 that it did not report unfavorable accident data to the government as mandated by law. TEPCO also admitted that it had falsified data in two hundred cases. In 2007, the company revealed yet more unreported accidents ("Tōden Genpatsu No Sōchikoshōwo Inpei" 2007).

3. For example, a CRMO in western Japan had noticed several problems with their detector, such as changes in the results over a course of several hours: The detected level of contamination tended to taper off and then rise again later. If a sample had a high level of potassium, the detector tended to falsely identify it as radioactive cesium. The staff reported these problems to the manufacturer, who was able to fix them. Also, CRMOs have helped tweak detectors in response to practical needs emerging from the reality of testing. For instance, a CRMO in the Tokyo metropolitan area has many volunteers who are housewives. They wanted to be able to monitor the testing process without staying at the center for hours, and they asked the software company to help them do so; the company developed a way to enable twenty-four-hour monitoring from the volunteers' homes.

4. The "strawberry complex" (*ichigo danchi*) was built in the towns of Watari and Yamamoto in Miyagi Prefecture after the disaster. These towns had already been famous for their strawberry farms, but the government reconstruction plan was not simply to go back to the predisaster state. Unlike the preaccident farms, the new strawberry complex utilizes aquaponics. While this might sound like a story of successful reconstruction, it entails various problems. Many farmers who used to grow strawberries complain that the strawberries from the factory taste different and are not as good as the ones they used to grow in soil. They have had a hard time adjusting to the new cultivation methods, and some complain that there is no longer room for creativity ("Ichigodanchikeikaku Ashibumi" 2012). The cost of growing with aquaponics is also much higher, and the system is vulnerable to damage in severe weather.

5. These incidents forced an international human rights group, Human Rights Watch, and other nonprofit organizations to request a visit by the UN Special Rapporteurs of Human Rights, including Anand Grover (Human Rights Now 2011a). Citing the examples above and others, he expressed grave concerns about the government's disregard of people's basic rights to health.

6. Studies such as one by Tsutsui, Muramatsu, and Higashino (2013) suggest that the Japanese norm of filial obligation in which daughters-in-law care for seniors is changing. However, even in their sample, a significant portion of primary care givers (more than 70 percent) were women.

Conclusion

1. This observation is echoed by studies of civic organizations in the United States. In their discussion on civil society and its political possibilities, sociologists Paul Lichterman and Nina Eliasoph (2014) point out that the nature of NGOs and civil society groups varies and that equating all of them unproblematically with civil society would be misleading. Even within NGOs, actions can oscillate between civic-minded and non-civic-minded. Attention to actual practices is also important in the context of NGO-ization, where NGOs are increasingly geared toward substituting for the state in social service provision rather than enabling political participation by citizens (Alvarez 2009; Bayat 2013). To find politics, it is necessary to ask what kinds of practices people are engaged with.

REFERENCES

Abe, Shinzo. 2014. "Policy Speech by Prime Minister Shinzo Abe to the 186th Session of the Diet." Prime Minister of Japan and His Cabinet, January 24. http://japan.kantei.go.jp/96_abe/statement/201401/24siseihousin_e.html.

"Abe Shushō Konkyo No Nai Fūhyō Ni Kunitoshite Zenryokude Taiō" [Prime Minister Abe, "The state will respond to baseless Fuhyo full force"]. 2014. *Sankei Shinbun*, May 17.

Adams, Vincanne, Michelle Murphy, and Adele E. Clarke. 2009. "Anticipation: Technoscience, Life, Affect, Temporality." *Subjectivity* 28 (1): 246–65.

Aegerter, Irene. 1989. "Women and Nuclear Power." IAEA. http://www.iaea.org/inis/collection/NCLCollectionStore/_Public/36/011/36011040.pdf.

Aeon Co. 2011. "Strengthening the Testing System with "Zero" Radioactive Materials in Stores." http://www.aeon.info/news/2011_2/pdf/111108R_1.pdf.

Agamben, Giorgio. 1998. *Homo Sacer: Sovereignty and Bare Life*. Stanford, CA: Stanford University Press.

Aldrich, Daniel P. 2010. *Site Fights: Divisive Facilities and Civil Society in Japan and the West*. Ithaca, NY: Cornell University Press.

———. 2013. "Rethinking Civil Society–State Relations in Japan after the Fukushima Accident." *Polity* 45 (2): 249–64.

Aldrich, D. P., and M. Dusinberre. 2011. "Hatoko Comes Home: Civil Society and Nuclear Power in Japan." *Journal of Asian Studies* 70 (3): 1–23.

Alexy, Allison. 2011. "Intimate Dependence and Its Risks in Neoliberal Japan." *Anthropological Quarterly* 84 (4): 895–917.

Alkon, Alison Hope, and Julian Agyeman. 2011. *Cultivating Food Justice: Race, Class, and Sustainability*. Cambridge, MA: MIT Press.

Allen, Patricia. 2007. *Together at the Table*. Philadelphia: Penn State Press.

Allison, Anne. 1996. "Producing Mothers." In *Re-Imaging Japanese Women*, edited by Anne Imamura, 135–55. Berkeley: University of California Press.

————. 2012. "Ordinary Refugees: Social Precarity and Soul in 21st Century Japan." *Anthropological Quarterly* 85 (2): 345–70.

Alvarez, Sonia E. 2009. "Beyond NGO-ization: Reflections from Latin America." *Development* 52 (2): 175–84.

Andō Jyun. 2014. "Genpatsu Ene Mondai Katariaujoseitachi Kaigaito Renkeimo" [Women discussing nuclear energy issue, collaboration with overseas]. *Nihon Keizai Shinbun*, June 21. http://www.nikkei.com/article/DGXNASDZ170K9 _Y4A610C1X93000/.

Ando, Takemasa. 2014. *Japan's New Left Movements: Legacies for Civil Society*. London: Routledge.

Aoyanagi Mami. 2012. "Heiwakenkyūkara Sotsugenpatu Undō E" [From peace studies to antinuclear movement]. *Okāsan Gyōkaishinbun*, January.

Apple, Rima D. 1996. *Vitamania: Vitamins in American Culture*. New Brunswick, NJ: Rutgers University Press.

Apter, David E., and Nagayo Sawa. 1984. *Against the State: Politics and Social Protest in Japan*. Cambridge, MA: Harvard University Press.

Araki Hitoshi. 2002. *Fūdo Shisutemu No Chirigakuteki Kenkyū* [Geography of food systems]. Tokyo: Taimeido.

Association for Future's Creation of Tamura and Children. n.d. http://www. たむら .jp/tamuramirai.html. Accessed August 1, 2014.

Association to Protect Children from Radiation in Yokohama. 2011. "Kōhō Yokohama Hōshasentokushūgō No Kaishū Oyobi Naiyōno Teisei Shazaiwo Motomeru Kōgiseimei" [Letter to demand revision and apology regarding Koho Yokohama's special issue on radiation]. September 16. http://yokohama-konan .info/kogiseimei.html.

Association to Protect Children in Shinagawa. 2014. "Shinagawaku, Zenkokudehajimete, Kyūshokushokuzaikensani Sutoronchiumukennsa Ga Kuwawarimasu" [First in the nation, in Shinagawa, school lunch food test will include strontium]. March 28. http://yashiochildren.wordpress.com.

Auyero, Javier, and Débora Alejandra Swistun. 2009. *Flammable: Environmental Suffering in an Argentine Shantytown*. Oxford: Oxford University Press.

Azuma Hirokatsu. 2011. "Hōshanō Osenmaiga Gisousarete Zenkokuni Baramakareteiru?" [The possibility of contaminated rice falsely labeled and sold nationwide?]. *Shokuhin to Kurashino Anzen*. http://alter.gr.jp/Preview.aspx?id =8342&cls=.

Baba Nobuhiko, and Ikeda Taishin, eds. 2012. *Joshi No Jidai* [The age of Joshi]. Tokyo: Seidosha.

Bäckstrand, Karin. 2004. "Scientisation vs. Civic Expertise in Environmental Governance: Eco-Feminist, Eco-Modern and Post-Modern Responses." *Environmental Politics* 13 (4): 695–714.

Bandazhevskaya, G. S., V. B. Nesterenko, V. I. Babenko, I. V. Babenko, T. V. Yerkovich, and Y. I. Bandazhevsky. 2004. "Relationship between Caesium (137Cs) Load,

Cardiovascular Symptoms, and Source of Food in 'Chernobyl' Children—Preliminary Observations after Intake of Oral Apple Pectin." *Swiss Medical Weekly* 134 (49–50): 725–29.

Bank of Japan. 2013. "Fukushimaken Ni Okeru Nōgyōno Genjō to Kadai" [Status quo and challenges facing Fukushima agriculture]. http://www3.boj.or.jp /fukushima/hoka/nougyou.pdf.

Barrett, Brendan F. D., ed. 2005. *Ecological Modernisation and Japan*. New York: Routledge.

Barton, Allen H. 1969. *Communities in Disaster: A Sociological Analysis of Collective Stress Situations*. Garden City, NY: Doubleday.

Bayat, Asef. 2013. *Life as Politics: How Ordinary People Change the Middle East*. Palo Alto, CA: Stanford University Press.

Beck, Ulrich. 1992. *Risk Society: Towards a New Modernity*. London: Sage.

Bekuredenegana. 2014. "Hōshanōkensa" [Radiation measurement]. February 16. http://beguredenega.com/archives/646.

"Bekurerufurī No Kodawari" [Why I care about becquerel free]. 2013. *VERY*, September, 224–26.

Blum, Elizabeth D. 2008. *Love Canal Revisited: Race, Class, and Gender in Environmental Activism*. Lawrence: University Press of Kansas.

Borovoy, Amy Beth. 2005. *The Too-Good Wife: Alcohol, Codependency, and the Politics of Nurturance in Postwar Japan*. Berkeley: University of California Press.

Boudia, Soraya. 2007. "Global Regulation: Controlling and Accepting Radioactivity Risks." *History and Technology* 23 (4): 389–406.

Boudia, Soraya, and Nathalie Jas. 2014. *Powerless Science? Science and Politics in a Toxic World*. New York: Berghahn.

Brown, Mark B. 2009. *Science in Democracy: Expertise, Institutions, and Representation*. Cambridge, MA: MIT Press.

Brown, Phil. 1992. "Popular Epidemiology and Toxic Waste Contamination: Lay and Professional Ways of Knowing." *Journal of Health and Social Behavior* 33 (3): 267–81.

———. 1993. "When the Public Knows Better: Popular Epidemiology." *Environment* 35 (8): 16–21.

Brown, Wendy. 2005. *Edgework: Critical Essays on Knowledge and Politics*. Princeton, NJ: Princeton University Press.

Burchell, Graham. 1996. "Liberal Government and Techniques of the Self." In *Foucault and Political Reason*, edited by Andrew Barry, Thomas Osborne, and Nikolas Rose, 19–36. Chicago: University of Chicago Press.

Cabinet Office. 2008. *Shokuikuhakusho* [Food education white paper]. Tokyo: Government of Japan.

———. 2011. "Press Conference by Prime Minister Yoshihiko Noda." Speeches and Statements by the Prime Minister, December 16. http://japan.kantei.go.jp/noda /statement/201112/16kaiken_e.html.

———. 2013a. *Shokuikuhakusho* [Food education white paper]. Tokyo: Government of Japan. http://www8.cao.go.jp/syokuiku/data/whitepaper/2013/book/html/sho2_03_03.html.

———. 2013b. "Presentation by Prime Minister Shinzo Abe at the 125th Session of the International Olympic Committee (IOC)." Speeches and Statements by the Prime Minister, September 7. http://japan.kantei.go.jp/96_abe/statement/201309/07ioc_presentation_e.html.

———. 2013c. "Address by Prime Minister Shinzo Abe, at the Sixty-Eighth Session of the General Assembly of the United Nations." Speeches and Statements by the Prime Minister, September 26. http://japan.kantei.go.jp/96_abe/statement/201309/26generaldebate_e.html.

———. 2014a. "Chiikino Keizai 2013" [Regional economy 2013]. Government of Japan. http://www5.cao.go.jp/j-j/cr/cr13/chr13_index.html.

———. 2014b. "Kōreishakaihakusho" [White paper on aging society]. Government of Japan. http://www8.cao.go.jp/kourei/whitepaper/w-2014/zenbun/s1_1_2.html.

Cavasin, Nathalie. 2008. "Citizen Activism and the Nuclear Industry in Japan: After the Tokai Village Disaster." In *Local Environmental Movements: A Comparative Study of the United States and Japan*, edited by Pradyumna Karan and Unryu Suganuma, 65–73. Lexington: University Press of Kentucky.

Centemeri, Laura. 2014. "What Kind of Knowledge Is Needed about Toxicant-Related Health Issues? Some Lessons Drawn from the Seveso Dioxin Case." In *Powerless Science? Science and Politics in a Toxic World*, edited by Soraya Boudia and Nathalie Jas, 134–51. New York: Berghahn.

Chōfu City. 2013. "Gakkōkyūshokuno Shokuzaini Kansuru Jizen No Hōshanōsokuteini Tsuiteno Chinjō" [Petition regarding prior radiation measurement of school food]. http://www.city.chofu.tokyo.jp/www/contents/1385438684052/simple/tinjyou_45.pdf.

Consumer Affairs Agency. 2013. *Fūhyōhigai Nikansuru Shōhishachōsa No Kekkatou Nitsuite* [Results of consumer survey on Fūhyōhigai]. Tokyo: Consumer Affairs Agency. http://www.caa.go.jp/safety/pdf/130311kouhyou_1.pdf.

Cooke, Bill, and Uma Kothari. 2001. *Participation: The New Tyranny?* London: Zed.

Corburn, Jason. 2005. *Street Science: Community Knowledge and Environmental Health Justice*. Cambridge, MA: MIT Press.

Daston, Lorraine. 2000. *Biographies of Scientific Objects*. Chicago: University of Chicago Press.

———. 2008. "On Scientific Observation." *Isis* 99 (1): 97–110.

Davies, Catriona. 2013. "The Woman Powering Japan's Nuclear Hopes Post-Fukushima." *CNN*, February 5. http://edition.cnn.com/2013/02/05/business/lady-judge-fukushima-japan-nuclear/.

Dean, Mitchell. 2002. "Liberal Government and Authoritarianism." *Economy and Society* 31 (1): 37–61.

"Dentōkōgei Ni 'Kawaii' Wo Fukikomu" [Revitalizing traditional crafts with cute-
ness]. 2014. *Senken Shinbun*, June 6. http://www.senken.co.jp/news/fashion-
buisnes-future-fukushima-goods/.

Dewey, John. 1999. "Search for the Public." In *The Science of Public Policy: Policy
Analysis*, edited by Tadao Miyakawa, 8–25. New York: Taylor and Francis.

Dolhinow, Rebecca. 2014. *Jumble of Needs: Women's Activism and Neoliberalism in the Colonias of the Southwest*. Minneapolis: University of Minnesota
Press.

Dudden, Alexis. 2012. "The Ongoing Disaster." *Journal of Asian Studies* 71 (2):
345–59.

Duggan, Lisa. 2012. *The Twilight of Equality? Neoliberalism, Cultural Politics, and
the Attack on Democracy*. Boston: Beacon.

Ehrenreich, Barbara. 2001. "Welcome to Cancerland." *Harper's*, November,
43–51.

Endo Kazuyuki, and Michimasa Matsumoto. 2012. "Shinsaifukkōni Muketa
Michinoekino Genjō to Kadai" [The present and problems of "Michi-No-Eki"
for postdisaster reconstruction]. *Nihon Toshigakkai Nenpo* 45. researchmap.
jp/?action=cv_download_main&upload_id=38725.

Endo Yasuo. 2012. *Genpatsujiko to Shokuhin Anzen* [Nuclear reactor accident and
food safety]. Tokyo: Nōrintōkeishuppan.

England, K. V. L. 1994. "Getting Personal: Reflexivity, Positionality, and Feminist
Research." *Professional Geographer* 46 (1): 80–89.

Epstein, Steven. 1998. *Impure Science: AIDS, Activism, and the Politics of Knowledge*.
Berkeley: University of California Press.

Eschle, Catherine. 2013. "Gender and the Subject of (Anti)Nuclear Politics: Revisit-
ing Women's Campaigning against the Bomb." *International Studies Quarterly*
57 (4): 713–24.

ETHOS Fukushima. n.d. "ETHOStte Nani?" [What is ETHOS?]. https://docs.google
.com/document/d/15SldUQh3M9giLv5B8NB-XzWTFQFwZSBlIFsRu_xojwI
/edit?hl=ja. Accessed June 2, 2014.

Farseta, Diane. 2008. "The Campaign to Sell Nuclear." *Bulletin of the Atomic Scientists* 64 (4): 38–56.

Ferber, Marianne A., and Julie A. Nelson. 2009. *Beyond Economic Man: Feminist
Theory and Economics*. Chicago: University of Chicago Press.

Fischer, Edward F., ed. 2008. *Indigenous Peoples, Civil Society, and the Neo-Liberal
State in Latin America*. New York: Berghahn.

Fischer, Frank. 2000. *Citizens, Experts, and the Environment: The Politics of Local
Knowledge*. Durham, NC: Duke University Press.

Fisheries Agency. n.d. http://www.jfa.maff.go.jp/j/housyanou/pdf/1410_kousin.pdf.
Accessed May 19, 2014.

Flynn, James, Paul Slovic, and Chris K. Mertz. 1994. "Gender, Race, and Perception
of Environmental Health Risks." *Risk Analysis* 14 (6): 1101–8.

Food Safety Commission. 2012. "Shokuhin Anzen Monitā Kadaihōkoku" [Report on issues from food safety monitors]. http://www.fsc.go.jp/monitor/2403moni-kadai-kekka.pdf.

Foodwatch. 2011. *Calculated Fatalities from Radiation.* https://www.foodwatch.org/uploads/tx_abdownloads/files/fw_report_CalculatedFatalitiesfromRadiation 11_2011.pdf.

Foucault, Michel. 1979. *Discipline and Punish: The Birth of the Prison.* New York: Vintage.

Fraser, Nancy. 1997. *Justice Interruptus: Critical Reflections on the "Postsocialist" Condition.* Oxford: Cambridge University Press.

———. 2013. "How Feminism Became Capitalism's Handmaiden—and How to Reclaim It." *Guardian,* October 14.

Freudenburg, W. R., and S. K. Pastor. 2005. "Public Responses to Technological Risks." *Sociological Quarterly* 33 (3): 389–412.

Frickel, S., S. Gibbon, J. Howard, J. Kempner, G. Ottinger, and D. J. Hess. 2010. "Undone Science: Charting Social Movement and Civil Society Challenges to Research Agenda Setting." *Science, Technology and Human Values* 35 (4): 444–73.

Fricker, Miranda. 2007. *Epistemic Injustice: Power and the Ethics of Knowing.* Oxford: Oxford University Press.

Fujita Hideo. 1984. "Nihon Ni Okeru PTA No Rekishi" [History of PTA in Japan]. *Risshodaigaku Bungakubu Kenkyukiyo* 1: 79–119.

"Fukushimagenpatsujiko Tokuteihinankaijode Teiso" [Suing government for lifting evacuation order after the Fukushima nuclear accident]. 2015. *Mainichi Shinbun,* April 17.

"Fukushimakarano Hinansha, Jinkenkyūsai Mōshitate Nyūenkyohinadono Fūhyōhigai" [Evacuees from Fukushima requesting human rights protection, victim of Fūhyōhigai]. 2012. *Mainichi Shinbun,* March 3.

"Fukushimakensanhinkawanai 30%" [Thirty percent responding they don't buy Fukushima food]. 2014. *Fukushima Minyu,* February 13. http://www.47news .jp/news/2014/02/post_20140213165704.html.

"Fukushima Kyōdō Shinryōjo Wo Kaisetsu" [Opening of the Fukushima Community Clinic]. 2013. *Weekly Zenshin,* January 1. http://www.zenshin.org/f_zenshin/f _back_no13/f2566sm.htm.

"Fukushima No Kikankijyun Hinanshazōwo Osorete Kyōkasezu Minshuseikenji" [Fukushima standards for returning were not strengthed, fearing increase in evacuees]. 2013. *Asahi Shinbun,* May 25. http://www.asahi.com/national/up date/0525/TKY201305250024.html.

Fukushima Prefecture. 2014. "Fukushimaken No Kōreishano Kazu" [The number of seniors in Fukushima Prefecture]. http://www.pref.fukushima.lg.jp /sec/11045b/16903.html.

Fukushima Prefecture and Fukushima Medical University. 2013. *Kōjōsenkensano Kekkanitsuite* [Results of thyroid cancer screening]. http://fukushima-mimamori .jp/thyroid-examination/media/pdf_resultsnotice_a.pdf.

"Gakkōkyūshoku No Shijōkibo" [Market size of school lunch]. 2008. *Gakko Kyūshoku*, July 10. http://gakkyu-news.net/jp/070/post_369.html.

"Garekishorihantainiwa 'Damare' Ishiharatochiji 'Minnanokyōryoku Hitsuyō'" ["Shut up" says Tokyo Governor Ishihara to opposition to debris, "Everyone needs to cooperate"]. 2011. *Sankei Shinbun*, November 4. http://sankei.jp.msn .com/politics/news/111104/lcl11110421490000-n1.htm.

Garon, Sheldon. 1998. *Molding Japanese Minds: The State in Everyday Life*. Princeton, NJ: Princeton University Press.

"Genbokuhoshishītake Kyūshokuriyō Kakudai Suishin" [Promoting the use of shiitake mushrooms in school lunches]. 2014. *Japan Agricultural Newspaper*, January 18.

Gender Equality Bureau. 2015. *Women and Men in Japan 2015*. Tokyo: Cabinet Office. http://www.gender.go.jp/english_contents/pr_act/pub/pamphlet/women -and-men15/.

George, Timothy S. 2001. *Minamata: Pollution and the Struggle for Democracy in Postwar Japan*. Cambridge, MA: Harvard University Press.

Ghaziani, Amin. 2008. *The Dividends of Dissent: How Conflict and Culture Work in Lesbian and Gay Marches on Washington*. Chicago: University of Chicago Press.

Gibbs, Lois Marie, and Murray Levine. 1982. *Love Canal: My Story*. Albany: State University of New York Press.

Gieryn, Thomas F. 1983. "Boundary-Work and the Demarcation of Science from Non-Science: Strains and Interests in Professional Ideologies of Scientists." *American Sociological Review* 48 (6): 781–95.

Glenn, Evelyn Nakano. 2000. "Creating a Caring Society." *Contemporary Sociology* 29 (1): 84–94.

González, A. J. 2012. "The Recommendations of the ICRP Vis-à-Vis the Fukushima Dai-Ichi NPP Accident Aftermath." *Journal of Radiological Protection* 32 (1): N1.

"Gōrikatsūchi" [Decree on rationalization]. 1999. *Gakkō Kyūshoku*, February. http://gakkyu-news.net/jp/010/011/post_58.html.

Gottlieb, Robert, and Anupama Joshi. 2010. *Food Justice*. Cambridge, MA: MIT Press.

Government of Japan. 2012. "Shokuhinchūno Hōshasei Busshitsuno Shinkijyunchi" [New standards for radioactive materials in food]. *Seifu Intānetto Terebi*. http://nettv.gov-online.go.jp/prg/prg6885.html.

———. 2013. *Fukushimadaiichigenshiryokuhatsudensho No Jiko Kara Ninen: Shokuhinchūno Hōshaseibusshitsu Wa Ima Dōnatteruno?* [Two years from the Fukushima no. 1 nuclear reactor accident: What is the state of radioactive materials in food?]. http://nettv.gov-online.go.jp/prg/prg8196.html.

Great East Japan Earthquake Reconstruction Headquarters. 2011. "Higashinihondaishinsai Karano Fukkō No Kihonhōshin" [Basic guidelines in response to

the Great East Japan Earthquake]. http://www.reconstruction.go.jp/topics
/doc/20110729houshin.pdf.

Greenpeace Japan. 2013a. "Dai21kai Chōsa" [Twenty-first survey]. http://www
.greenpeace.org/japan/ja/campaign/monitoring/21st/.

Greenpeace Japan. 2013b. "Shokuhinhōshanochōsa Dai 13kaime" [Thirteenth survey of radiation contamination of food]. April 23. http://www.greenpeace.org
/japan/fss13/.

Griffin, Penny. 2007. "Sexing the Economy in a Neo-Liberal World Order: Neo-
Liberal Discourse and the (Re)Production of Heteronormative Heterosexual-
ity." *British Journal of Politics and International Relations* 9 (2): 220–38.

Grove, Kevin. 2014. "Agency, Affect, and the Immunological Politics of Disaster
Resilience." *Environment and Planning D: Society and Space* 32 (2): 240–56.

Guthman, J. 2003. "Fast Food/Organic Food: Reflexive Tastes and the Making of
'Yuppie Chow.'" *Social and Cultural Geography* 4 (1): 45–58.

"Gyūnyūnomazu Beihan Wa Jisan" [Not drinking milk and bringing rice from
home]. 2013. *Yomiuri Shinbun*, February 4.

Hacking, Ian. 2002. *Historical Ontology*. Cambridge, MA: Harvard University Press.

Harding, Sandra G. 1991. *Whose Science? Whose Knowledge? Thinking from Women's
Lives*. Ithaca, NY: Cornell University Press.

Hasegawa, Koichi. 1995. "A Comparative Study of Social Movements in the Post-
Nuclear Energy Era in Japan and the United States." *International Journal of
Japanese Sociology* 4 (1): 21–36.

Hawkesworth, Mary E. 2001. "Democratization: Reflections on Gendered Dislo-
cations in the Public Sphere." In *Gender, Globalization, and Democratization*,
edited by Rita Mae Kelly, Jane H. Bayes, Mary E. Hawkesworth, and Brigitte
Young, 223–36. Lanham, MD: Rowman and Littlefield.

Health Protection Agency. 2009. "Application of the 2007 Recommendations of the
ICRP to the UK." London: Health Protection Agency. http://webarchive.nation-
alarchives.gov.uk/20140714084352/http://www.hpa.org.uk/webc/hpawebfile
/hpaweb_c/1246519364845.

Hecht, Gabrielle. 2012. *Being Nuclear: Africans and the Global Uranium Trade*.
Cambridge, MA: MIT Press.

Hess, D. J. 2007. *Alternative Pathways in Science and Industry: Activism, Innovation,
and the Environment in an Era of Globalization*. Cambridge, MA: MIT Press.

———. 2009. "The Potentials and Limitations of Civil Society Research: Getting
Undone Science Done." *Sociological Inquiry* 79 (3): 306–27.

Hidaka Noboru. 2012. "Kimin" [Abandoned people]. In *Datsugenpatu Shizen
Enerugī 218nin Shisyū* [Farewell to nuclear, welcome to renewable energy: A
collection of poems by 218 poets], 53. Tokyo: Coal-Sack.

High, Casey, Ann H. Kelly, and Jonathan Mair. 2012. *The Anthropology of Ignorance:
An Ethnographic Approach*. London: Palgrave Macmillan.

Holdgrun, Phoebe, and Barbara Holthus. 2014. "Gender and Political Participation in Post-3/11 Japan." *German Institute for Japanese Studies Working
Paper Series* 14 (3). http://www.dijtokyo.org/publications/WP1403_Hold
gruen_Holthus.pdf.

Holloway, Susan D. 2010. *Women and Family in Contemporary Japan.* Cambridge:
Cambridge University Press.

Holthus, Barbara, and Hiromi Tanaka. 2013. "Parental Well-Being and the Sexual
Division of Household Labor: A New Look at Gendered Families in Japan."
Asiatische Studien 67 (2): 401–28.

Honda, Hiroshi. 2003. "Nihon No Genshiryokuseijikatei (4): Rengōkeisei to
Funsōkanri" [Process of Japanese nuclear policy: Coalition making and conflict
resolution]. *Hokkaido University Legal Journal* 54 (1): 394–462.

Honma Masato. 2007. *Monsutā Pearento* [Monster parents]. Tokyo: Chukei
Shuppan.

Honma Ryu. 2013. *Genpatsukōkoku* [Nuclear PR]. Tokyo: Aki Shobō.

Hōshanōbusshitsu Kiseichigoe Fukushimakenyasai 43pinchu 25hin [Twenty-five
out of forty-three Fukushima vegetables above radioactive standards]. 2011.
Mainichi Shinbun, March 31.

"Hōshanōosen No Gakkōkyūshoku Hahaoyatachiwa Genkai Ni Kiteiru" [Radiation
contamination of school lunches exhausts mothers' patience]. 2014. *Tanaka
Ryusaku Journal,* January 30. http://tanakaryusaku.jp/2011/08/0002754.

"Hōshanō Towa" [What is radiation brain]. 2011. *Nico Nico Pedia,* December 30.
http://dic.nicovideo.jp/a/%E6%94%BE%E5%B0%84%E8%84%B3.

"Hōshasenseshiumu Osengyū" [Beef contaminated by radioactive cesium]. 2011.
Japan Business Press, October 7. http://jbpress.ismedia.jp/articles/-/24624
?page=6.

Hoshi, Masaharu, Yuri O. Konstantinov, Tatiana Y. Evdeeva, Andrey I. Kovalev,
Alexandr S. Aksenov, Natalya V. Koulikova, Hitoshi Sato, et al. 2000. "Radioce-
sium in Children Residing in the Western Districts of the Bryansk Oblast from
1991–1996." *Health Physics* 79 (2): 182–86.

Human Rights Now. 2011a. "Human Rights Violation after Fukushima Disaster
and Great East Japan Earthquake: A Country Visit to Japan by UN Special
Rapporteurs." July 26. http://hrn.or.jp/eng/activity/area/japan/request-of-a
-country-visit-to-japan-by-un-special-rapporteurs/.

———. 2011b. "Fukushima, Koriyama Chōsahōkokusho" [Report on Fukushima
and Koriyama]. http://hrn.or.jp/activity/.

———. 2013. "Kokurenkagakuiinkai Ni Taisuru Seimei" [Comments on the
UNSCEAR]. October 22. http://hrn.or.jp/activity/topic/post-235/.

Hurnung, Jeffrey W. 2011. "The Risks of 'Disaster Nationalism.'" PacNet #34, July 13.
Center for Strategic and International Studies. http://csis.org/publication/pacnet
-34-risks-disaster-nationalism.

Hymans, Jacques E. C. 2010. "East Is East, and West Is West? Currency Iconography as Nation-Branding in the Wider Europe." *Political Geography* 29 (2): 97–108.

"IAEA Urges Japan to Give Public a Dose of Reality on Decontamination Work." 2013. *Asahi Shinbun*, October 23. http://ajw.asahi.com/article/0311disaster /fukushima/AJ201310230076.

"Ichigodanchikeikaku Ashibumi" [Challenges to the plan for the Strawberry Complex]. 2012. *Livedoor News*, April 14. http://news.livedoor.com/article/detail /6467923/.

ICRP. 2012a. "Conclusions and Recommendations of the Second Dialogue Meeting." Ottawa: ICRP. http://www.icrp.org/docs/Dialogue-2-Conclusions.pdf.

———. 2012b. "Third Dialogue on the Rehabilitation of Living Conditions after the Fukushima Accident." Ottawa: ICRP. http://www.icrp.org/docs/dialogue -3E.pdf.

Ikeda Nobuo. 2013. "Yamamoto Taro Wa Chūkaku-Ha No Shienkōhō" [Yamamoto Taro endorsed by Chūkaku-Ha]. *Ikeda Nobuo Blog*, July 18. http://ikedanobuo .livedoor.biz/archives/51864901.html.

Imazato, Satoshi. 2008. "Under Two Globalizations: Progress in Social and Cultural Geography of Japanese Rural Areas, 1996–2006." *Geographical Review of Japan* 81 (5): 323–35.

Inoue Hiraku. 2012. "Hōshanōosen No Rekishito Shiminsokuteino Igi" [History of radiation contamination and the value of citizen measurement]. Toxic Watch, September 6. http://www.toxwatch.net/HP/houshanou_B/pdf/soku teinoigi1209.pdf.

Inter-Faith Forum for Review of National Nuclear Policy. 2012. "2012 Fukushima Zenkoku Shūkai Apīru" [Appeal at the 2012 national meeting in Fukushima]. http://gts.mukakumuhei.net/advocacy.htm#2012fukushimaappeal.

Inter-Parliamentary Union. 2014. "Women in National Parliaments." http://www .ipu.org/wmn-e/classif.htm.

Irwin, Alan. 1995. *Citizen Science: A Study of People, Expertise and Sustainable Development*. London: Routledge.

Ishibashi Suomi. 2007. "Watashino Sutekina Rōrumoderu" [My fantastic role model]. *Energy Review*, August, 29.

Ishii Miso Co. n.d. "Misoniyoru Hōshasenbōgyosayō to Ketsuatsuyokuseisayō Nitsuite" [On antiradiation protective function and blood pressure–lowering effects of miso]. *Science of Miso*. http://ishiimiso.com/miso/kono_9.html. Accessed May 15, 2014.

Ishii Takaaki. 2012. "Hōshanō, Ko Yue No Yami" [Radiation, darkness because of children]. *Agora*, January 21. http://agora-web.jp/archives/1424611.html.

Ishikawa Yuki. 2007. *Monsutāmazā* [Monster mothers]. Tokyo: Kobunsha.

"Itō-Yōkadō Osenutagaigyuwo 94tenpode Hanbai" [Itō-Yōkadō Sold Beef Suspected of Contamination at 94 Stores]. 2011. *Yomiuri Shinbun*, July 21.

Iwase Tadatsu. 2013. "Nihonkeizaino Genjō" [Reality and challenges of Japanese economy]. Ministry of Finance Policy Research Institute. https://www.mof.go .jp/pri/summary/kouen/kou021.pdf.

Jalbert, Kirk, Abby J. Kinchy, and Simona L. Perry. 2014. "Civil Society Research and Marcellus Shale Natural Gas Development: Results of a Survey of Volunteer Water Monitoring Organizations." *Journal of Environmental Studies and Sciences* 4: 78–86.

Japan Private Schools Education Institute. 2014. "Gakkosūnosuii" [Trends in the number of schools]. Tokyo. http://www.shigaku.or.jp/news/school.pdf.

Japan Scientists' Association. 2014. *Kokusaigenshiryokumura* [International nuclear village]. Tokyo: Godo Shuppan.

"Japan's Earthquake: Emperor Akihito 'Deeply Worried.'" 2011. *BBC News*, March 16. http://www.bbc.co.uk/news/world-asia-pacific-12755739.

Jaquette, Jane S., and Sharon L. Wolchik, eds. 1998. *Women and Democracy: Latin America and Central and Eastern Europe.* Baltimore, MD: Johns Hopkins University Press.

Jasanoff, Sheila. 2005. *Design on Nature: Science and Democracy in Europe and the United States.* Princeton, NJ: Princeton University Press.

Jen, Clare Ching. 2013. "How to Survive Contagion, Disease, and Disaster: The 'Masked Asian/American Woman' as Low-Tech Specter of Emergency Preparedness." *Feminist Formations* 25 (2): 107–28.

Jessop, Bob. 2002. "Liberalism, Neoliberalism, and Urban Governance: A State-Theoretical Perspective." *Antipode* 34 (3): 452–72.

Judge, Barbara. n.d. "Message from Lady Barbara Judge CBE, Deputy Chairman." Nuclear Reform Monitoring Committee. http://www.nrmc.jp/en/member/de tail/1224355_5228.html. Accessed June 22, 2014.

Kainuma Hiroshi. 2011. *Fukushimaron* [Theory of Fukushima]. Tokyo: Seidosha.

Kamiyama Michiko. 2013. "Shōhishachō No Fūhyōhigaini Kansuru Shōhishachōsano Kekkatō Nitsuite" [Consumer protection agency's results of survey of consumers regarding Fūhyo Higai]. Citizen's Committee to Monitor Food Safety, April 24. http://www.fswatch.org/2013/4-24.htm.

Kanda, Tomoko, Takako Nagai, and Daisuke Shinohara. 2011. "Questions to Corporations about Safety Responses." *Shūkan Asahi*, October 28.

Kansho Taeko. 1978. *Mada Maniaunorana* [If it is still not too late]. Tokyo: Jiyusha.

Karaki Hideaki. 2011. "Kiseichi Wa Anzen to Kiken No Kyōkai Dewa Arimasen" [Standards are not a boundary between safety and danger]. *Koho Yokohama*, September.

Kataoka Terumi. 2012. *Ima, Inochiwo Mamoru* [Protect life now]. Tokyo: Nihon Kirisuto Kyodan Shuppan.

Kawahara Kazue. 2012. "Joshi No Imisayo" [Function and meaning of Joshi]. In *Joshi No Jidai* [The age of Joshi], edited by Nobuhiko Baba and Taishin Ikeda, 17–36. Tokyo: Seikyusha.

Kelsky, Karen. 2001. *Women on the Verge*. Durham, NC: Duke University Press.

Kennelly, Jacqueline. 2009. "Good Citizen/Bad Activist: The Cultural Role of the State in Youth Activism." *Review of Education, Pedagogy, and Cultural Studies* 31 (2–3): 127–49.

Kerkvliet, Benedict J. 1990. *Everyday Politics in the Philippines: Class and Status Relations in a Central Luzon Village*. Berkeley: University of California Press.

Kimura, Aya H. 2008. "Who Defines Babies' Needs? The Scientization of Baby Food in Indonesia." *Social Politics: International Studies in Gender, State and Society* 15 (2): 232–60.

———. 2011. "Food Education as Food Literacy: Privatized and Gendered Food Knowledge in Contemporary Japan." *Agriculture and Human Values* 28 (4): 465–82.

———. 2013a. *Hidden Hunger: Gender and the Politics of Smarter Foods*. Ithaca, NY: Cornell University Press.

———. 2013b. "Standards as Hybrid Forum: Comparison of the Post-Fukushima Radiation Standards by a Consumer Cooperative, the Private Sector, and the Japanese Government." *International Journal of Sociology of Agriculture and Food* 20 (1): 11–29.

Kimura, Aya H., and Mima Nishiyama. 2008. "The Chisan-Chisho Movement: Japanese Local Food Movement and Its Challenges." *Agriculture and Human Values* 25 (1): 49–64.

Kinchy, Abby. 2012. *Seeds, Science, and Struggle: The Global Politics of Transgenic Crops*. Cambridge, MA: MIT Press.

King, Samantha. 2006. *Pink Ribbons, Inc.: Breast Cancer and the Politics of Philanthropy*. Minneapolis: University of Minnesota Press.

Kirasienne Shuppan, ed. 2011. *Nihonshokuga Anatawosukuu, Hōshanōdetokkusunokagiwa Nihonshokuni Atta* [Japanese food will save you—the key to radioactive detoxing lies in Japanese food]. Tokyo: Kirasienne Shuppan.

Kitahara Minori, and Pak Su Yi. 2014. *Okusamawa Aikoku* [Housewives' patriotism]. Tokyo: Kawade Shobo Shinsha.

Kitamura, Naoki. 2011. Kyūshoku ni tsukawareta fukushimakensangy ūniku shōsai kisainashi no nazo [Question of "no details" on Fukushima beef used in school lunches]. *Nikkan Spa*. August 20. http://nikkan-spa.jp/45434.

Kitsunai Kumi. 2006. "Hāto to Hāto No Kōryu Wo Kasanete" [Accumulating heart-to-heart exchanges]. *Genshiryoku Eye* 52 (2): 78–79.

Klawiter, Maren. 2008. *The Biopolitics of Breast Cancer: Changing Cultures of Disease and Activism*. Minneapolis: University of Minnesota Press.

Klein, Naomi. 2005. *The Rise of Disaster Capitalism*. DVD. National Emergency Training Center. http://www.pmpress.org/productsheets/pm_titles/risedisaster.pdf.

———. 2007. *The Shock Doctrine: The Rise of Disaster Capitalism*. London: Macmillan.

Kleinman, Daniel Lee. 2000. *Science, Technology, and Democracy*. Albany: State University of New York Press.

Kleinman, Daniel Lee, and Sainath Suryanarayanan. 2012. "Dying Bees and the Social Production of Ignorance." *Science, Technology and Human Values* 1 (1): 1–26.

Kobayashi, Yoshie. 2004. *Path toward Gender Equality: State Feminism in Japan*. London: Routledge.

Kodama Tatsuhiko. 2011. *Naibuhibakuno Shinjitsu* [The truth about internal radiation]. Tokyo: Gentosha.

"Kodomotachino Shokuno Anzenwo Tettei" [Ensuring safety of school lunches]. 2012. *Disaster Goods News*, June 10. http://www.disaster-goods.com/news _0838FOGXo.html.

Koertge, Noretta. 2005. "What Science Can Offer Contemporary Democracy." In *Scientific Values and Civic Virtues*, edited by Noretta Koertge, 3–4. Oxford: Oxford University Press.

Koide Goro. 2013. "Risuku Komyunikēshon" [Risk communication]. *Kagaku to Kogyo* [Chemistry and industry] 66 (6): 435–36.

Koide Hiroaki. 2011. *Genpatsu No Uso* [Lies of the nuclear power plants]. Tokyo: Fusosha.

Konosu Tadashi. 2004. "Seikabutsutorihikino Aitaikatokakakukeiseinokadai" [Aitai sales in fresh vegetables and fruits and the problem of price formation]. *Norinkinyu* 9: 22–33.

Kubo Jyunichi. 2012. "Shokuhin Ni Kansuru Risuku Komyunikēshon Shokuhincyūno Hōshaseibusshitsu Ni Kansuru Ikenkōkan" [Minutes of risk communication regarding food opinion exchange regarding radioactive materials in food]. Ehime, Japan, July 24. http://www.mhlw.go.jp/topics/bukyoku/iyaku/syoku -anzen/iken/dl/120420-1-ehime_5.pdf.

Kuchinskaya, Olga. 2014. *The Politics of Invisibility: Public Knowledge about Radiation Health Effects after Chernobyl*. Cambridge, MA: MIT Press.

"Kujyū Hibakujirikikensa" [Struggle to pay for radiation exposure measurement]. 2014. *Tokyo Shinbun*, April 22.

Kumasaka Hitomi. 2014. "Hontōni Fukushimadetottanoka to Kaigaikarautagaware-teiru Happy Fukushimaban Tōjōjinbutsuno Haikei" [Background of people appearing in Happy Fukushima version]. *Yahoo News*, June 8. http://bylines.news .yahoo.co.jp/kumasakahitomi/20140608-00036150/.

Kunihiro, Yoko. 2011. "The Politicization of Housewives." In *Transforming Japan: How Feminism and Diversity Are Making a Difference*, edited by Kumiko Fujimura-Fanselow, 360–75. New York: Feminist Press.

"Kyūshokuni Hōshanōkijyun, 1kiro 40 Bekureru" [Radiation standard in school lunches at 40 Bq/kg]. 2011. *Asahi Shinbun*, December 1. http://www.asahi.com /special/10005/TKY201111300868.html.

"Kyūshokuniyoru Naibuhibakukara Kodomotachiwo Mamoruameni" [In order to protect children from internal radiation associated with school lunches.]" January 30, 2014. A blog by a Yokosuka City Council Member, Fujino Hideaki. http://www.hide-fujino.com/blog/2014/01/30/17662.

"Kyūshokuno Shokuzai Hōshanō Sokutei Shutoken No Jichitai" [Measuring radiation in school lunch food by municipal governments in the metropolitan area]. 2011. *Asahi Shinbun*, July 6. http://www.asahi.com/special/10005/TKY201107050804.html.

"Lady Barbara Judge San to No Tōku Sesshon" [Talk session with Lady Barbara Judge]. 2013. *Love You!*, April 27. http://denisaya.jugem.jp/?eid=112.

Lang, Sabina. 2001. "The NGOization of Feminism." In *Transitions, Environments, Translations: Feminisms in International Politics*, edited by J. W. Scott, C. Kaplan, and D. Keats, 101–20. New York: Routledge.

Lave, Rebecca. 2012. "Neoliberalism and the Production of Environmental Knowledge." *Environment and Society: Advances in Research* 3 (1): 19–38.

LeBlanc, R. M. 1999. *Bicycle Citizens: The Political World of the Japanese Housewife*. Berkeley: University of California Press.

Lebra, Takie Sugiyama. 1976. *Japanese Patterns of Behaviour*. Honolulu: University of Hawai'i Press.

Levine, Susan. 2010. *School Lunch Politics: The Surprising History of America's Favorite Welfare Program*. Princeton, NJ: Princeton University Press.

Lichterman, Paul, and Nina Eliasoph. 2014. "Civic Action." *American Journal of Sociology* 120 (3): 798–863.

Lindee, M. Susan. 2008. *Suffering Made Real: American Science and the Survivors at Hiroshima*. Chicago: University of Chicago Press.

Little, Mark P., Maria Blettner, John D. Boice Jr., Bryn A. Bridges, Elisabeth Cardis, Monty W. Charles, Florent de Vathaire, Richard Doll, Kenzo Fujimoto, and Dudley Goodhead. 2004. "Potential Funding Crisis for the Radiation Effects Research Foundation." *Lancet* 364 (9434): 557–58.

Lochard, Jacques. 2012. "The Fukushima Dialogue Initiative." Presented at the Seventieth CRPPH Meeting, Paris, March 21–23. https://docs.google.com/file/d/0BxqSmDmQ78xCLTVWejZaakNSc3VlZktpX1ZVVUdRUQ/edit.

Lochard, J., E. Bogdevitch, E. Gallego, P. Hedemann-Jensen, A. McEwan, A. Nisbet, A. Oudiz, P. Strand, A. Janssens, and T. Lazo. 2009. "Application of the Commission's Recommendations to the Protection of People Living in Long-Term Contaminated Areas after a Nuclear Accident or a Radiation Emergency." *Annals of the ICRP* 39 (3).

Lora-Wainwright, Anna. 2013. "The Inadequate Life: Rural Industrial Pollution and Lay Epidemiology in China." *China Quarterly* 214 (June): 302–20.

Luft, Rachel E. 2009. "Beyond Disaster Exceptionalism: Social Movement Developments in New Orleans after Hurricane Katrina." *American Quarterly* 61 (3): 499–527.

Mackie, Vera C. 2003. *Feminism in Modern Japan: Citizenship, Embodiment and Sexuality*. Cambridge: Cambridge University Press.

Makishita Keiki. 2013. *Hōshanō Osen to Gakkōkyūshoku* [Radiation contamination and school lunches]. Tokyo: Iwanami Shoten.

Managhan, Tina. 2007. "Shifting the Gaze from Hysterical Mothers to 'Deadly Dads': Spectacle and the Anti-Nuclear Movement." *Review of International Studies* 33 (4): 637–54.

Marres, Noortje. 2007. "The Issues Deserve More Credit: Pragmatist Contributions to the Study of Public Involvement in Controversy." *Social Studies of Science* 37 (5): 759–80.

"Marudekakurekirishitan? Hōshanōrakkanha to Tatakau Hahaoyatachi" [Like hidden Christians? Mothers fighting against optimists about radiation]. 2013. *Aera*, September 26. http://dot.asahi.com/aera/2013092500036.html.

Matsunaga Kazuki. 2011a. "Fukenshutsunanoni Hōshanōnuki Shinan" [Advising anti-radiation although nondetectable?]. *Food Communication Compass*, June 30. http://www.foocom.net/column/editor/4420/.

———. 2011b. "Kenkōshokuhinde Gedoku Wo Shinjitewa Ikenai" [Don't believe in "detoxing by health foods"]. *Food Communication Compass*, July 9. http://www.foocom.net/column/editor/4494/.

———. 2012. "Tekiseishōhishakihan Wo Tsukurō: Okāsan No Tameno Shokunoanzen Kyōshitsu Kankō Ni Yosete" [Making good consumer practice: Upon the publication of "Food Safety Lessons for Mothers"]. *Food Communication Compass*, December 20. http://www.foocom.net/column/editor/8381/.

May, Todd. 2008. *The Political Thought of Jacques Rancière: Creating Equality*. University Park, PA: Penn State Press.

McDonald, Alan, and Holger Rogner. 2011. "IAEA Projects Slower Nuclear Growth after Fukushima." *IAEA News*, September 22. http://www.iaea.org/newscenter/news/2011/nuclgrowth.html.

McGray, Douglas. 2009. "Japan's Gross National Cool." *Foreign Policy*, November 11, 44–54.

McRobbie, Angela. 2007. "TOP GIRLS? Young Women and the Post-Feminist Sexual Contract 1." *Cultural Studies* 21 (4–5): 718–37.

———. 2009. *The Aftermath of Feminism: Gender, Culture and Social Change*. London: Sage.

Merton, Robert K. 1973. *The Sociology of Science: Theoretical and Empirical Investigations*. Chicago: University of Chicago Press.

"Minami-Soma Lambastes Government, TEPCO for Remaining Mum on Rice Contamination." 2014. *Asahi Shinbun*, July 15. http://ajw.asahi.com/article/0311disaster/fukushima/AJ201407150040.

Minashita Kiryu. 2013. *Joshikai 2.0* [Joshi Party 2.0]. Tokyo: NHK Shuppan.

Ministry of Agriculture, Forestry and Fisheries. 2014. "Heisei25nendo No Nōsanbutsu Ni Fukumareru Hōshaseiseshiumu Nōdo No Kensakekka" [Results of radioactive

cesium concentration in agricultural produce in FY 2013]. April 16. http://www
.maff.go.jp/j/kanbo/joho/saigai/s_chosa/H25gaiyo.html.

Ministry of Economics, Trade, and Industry. 2009. "Kankei Dētashū" [Related
data]. http://www.mext.go.jp/b_menu/shingi/gijyutu/gijyutu10/toushin/__ics
Files/afieldfile/2009/05/18/1260184_1.pdf.

Ministry of Education, Culture, Sports, Science and Technology. 2010. "Gakkō
Kyūshoku Jisshi Jōkyō Chōsa" [Survey of school lunch implementation]. http://
www.mext.go.jp/b_menu/toukei/chousa05/kyuushoku/kekka/k_detail/1320912
.htm.

———. 2011. "Shinendokarano Gakkōkyūshokuno Jisshini Atatteno Ryūitennitsuite"
[Points to be careful with in implementing school lunches for the new academic
year]. http://www.mext.go.jp/a_menu/saigaijohou/syousai/1304779.htm.

———. 2012. "Gakkōkyūshokuhi No Chōsyū Jōkyō Ni Kansuru Chōsano Kekka
Nitsuite" [Results of the survey on collection of school lunch fees]. http://www
.mext.go.jp/b_menu/houdou/24/04/1321085.htm.

Ministry of Health, Labor, and Welfare. 2011. "Hōshanō Osen Sareta Shokuhin No
Toriatsukaini Tsuite" [Handling of foods contaminated by radioactive materials].
http://www.mhlw.go.jp/stf/houdou/2r9852000001558e-img/2r9852000001559v
.pdf.

———. 2012. "Shokuhinchū No Hōshaseibusshitsuno Kensa Ni Tsuite" [On results
of radiation screening of foods]. https://www.fsc.go.jp/fsciis/.

———. 2013. "Shokuhinchūno Hōshaseibusshitsuno Taisakuto Genjō Ni Tsuite"
[Regarding status and the responses to radioactive materials in food]. http://
www.mhlw.go.jp/shinsai_jouhou/dl/20131025-1.pdf.

Ministry of Internal Affairs and Communications. 2012. "Higashinihondaishinsaigono
Wagakunino Sōjinkō No Ugoki" [Population trends after the Great East Japan
Earthquake]. Government of Japan. http://www.stat.go.jp/data/jinsui/2011np
/pdf/gaiyou.pdf.

Miyagi Prefecture Division of Agriculture, Forestry and Fisheries. 2012. "Tokyodenryoku Fukushimadaiichigenshiryokuhatsudenshojiko Ni Tomonau
Miyagiken No Nōrinsuisanbutsu Fūhyōhigaino Jittaihaaku" [Report on Fuhyo-
higai experienced by Miyagi's Agriculture, Forestry, and Fisheries due to the
accident at TEPCO Fukushima Daiichi nuclear power plant]. https://www.r
-info-miyagi.jp/site/wp-content/uploads/2012/09/34e401221f5864206387a0a0
af862a0a.pdf.

Mol, Arthur P. J. 2003. *Globalization and Environmental Reform: The Ecological
Modernization of the Global Economy*. Cambridge, MA: MIT Press.

Mollett, Sharlene, and Caroline Faria. 2013. "Messing with Gender in Feminist Political Ecology." *Geoforum* 45: 116–25.

Moodie, Megan. 2013. "Microfinance and the Gender of Risk: The Case of Kiva.org."
Signs: Journal of Women in Culture and Society 38 (2): 279–302.

Moore, Kelly, Daniel Lee Kleinman, David Hess, and Scott Frickel. 2011. "Science and Neoliberal Globalization: A Political Sociological Approach." *Theory and Society* 40 (5): 505–32.

Morgen, Sandra. 2002. *Into Our Own Hands: The Women's Health Movement in the United States, 1969–1990.* New Brunswick, NJ: Rutgers University Press.

Mori, Masako. 2014. *Comments by Minister of State for Consumer Affairs and Food Safety.* 13 vols. Tokyo.

Morioka, Rika. 2014. "Gender Difference in the Health Risk Perception of Radiation from Fukushima in Japan: The Role of Hegemonic Masculinity." *Social Science and Medicine* 107: 105–12.

Morita, Atsuro, Anders Blok, and Shuhei Kimura. 2013. "Environmental Infrastructures of Emergency: The Formation of a Civic Radiation Monitoring Map during the Fukushima Disaster." In *Nuclear Disaster at Fukushima Daiichi: Social, Political and Environmental Issues*, edited by Richard Hindmarsh, 78–96. New York: Routledge.

Morita Maki. 2011. "Shokuhin Anzen Iinkai Syūryōgo No Kishakaiken" [Press conference after the Food Safety Commission]. *Food Communication Compass*, July 31. http://www.foocom.net/secretariat/observer/4683/.

Morita Toshiya. 2012a. "Kyoto Shiminhōshanō Sokuteijo Ōpunnisaishite" [Upon the opening of Kyoto Citizen Radiation Measuring Station]. *Asunimukete*, April 8. http://blog.goo.ne.jp/tomorrow_2011/e/7115f820e164346c1ed9fba6dec977be.

———. 2012b. "Amerikaniyoru Naibuhibakukakushito RERF" [Internal radiation made invisible by the US and RERF]. *Asunimukete*, July 29. http://blog.goo.ne.jp/tomorrow_2011/e/c6a9b0ff6b1c6ed4c3a46c898a795724.

Morris-Suzuki, Tessa. 2014a. "Invisible Politics." *Humanities Australia* 5: 53–64.

———. 2014b. "Touching the Grass: Science, Uncertainty and Everyday Life from Chernobyl to Fukushima." *Science, Technology and Society* 19 (3): 331–62.

Mothers' Group to Investigate Early Radiation Exposure. 2013a. "Ninshikinochigaikara Umareta Bundan" [Schisms as a result of different understandings]. February 22. http://iwakinomama.jugem.jp/?eid=7.

———. 2013b. "Kazokunotameni Shakaino Nakade Ganbatteiru Otōsan E" [To fathers who are doing their best in society for their family]. May 9. http://iwakinomama.jugem.jp/?cid=19.

———. 2014. "Kodomowo Naibuhibakukara Mamorutame Gakkōkyūshokuno Shokuzaini Hairyowo Negauyōbōsho Wo Teishutsushimashita" [Submitted a petition to ask for care in school lunch food in order to protect children from internal radiation]. March 20. http://iwakinomama.jugem.jp/?page=4&cid=32.

Mukerji, Chandra. 1994. "The Political Mobilization of Nature in Seventeenth-Century French Formal Gardens." *Theory and Society* 23 (5): 651–77.

———. 2002. "Material Practices of Domination: Christian Humanism, the Built Environment, and Techniques of Western Power." *Theory and Society* 31 (1): 1–34.

———. 2009. *Impossible Engineering: Technology and Territoriality on the Canal Du Midi*. Princeton, NJ: Princeton University Press.

Murphy, Michelle. 2006. *Sick Building Syndrome and the Problem of Uncertainty: Environmental Politics, Technoscience, and Women Workers*. Durham, NC: Duke University Press.

———. 2012. *Seizing the Means of Reproduction: Entanglements of Feminism, Health, and Technoscience*. Durham, NC: Duke University Press.

My Town Fukushima. 2012. "11 Shichōson Chōka No Keiken, Kyūshokuno Hōshanō" [Eleven municipalities' experiences of the standard, contaminated school lunch]. September 17. http://blogs.yahoo.co.jp/kyomutekisonzairon/65915474.html.

Nagoya Seikatsu Kurabu. n.d. "Aichikensan Kyabetsu No Hōshanō Osen Wa Mondai Arimasen" [No radiation problem with Aichi cabbage]. http://3.nagoyasei katsuclub.com/?eid=25. Accessed October 27, 2014.

Nakagawa Yasuo. 1991. *Hōshasenhibaku No Rekishi* [History of radiation exposure]. Tokyo: Akashi Shoten.

Nakane, Chie. 1970. *Japanese Society*. Berkeley: University of California Press.

Nakano Masashi. 2014. *Ukeishakai Nippon* (The right-wing turn of Japan). Tokyo: Discover 21.

Naples, Nancy A. 2014. *Grassroots Warriors: Activist Mothering, Community Work, and the War on Poverty*. London: Routledge.

Negra, Diane. 2014. "Claiming Feminism: Commentary, Autobiography and Advice Literature for Women in the Recession." *Journal of Gender Studies* 23 (3): 275–86.

Nelson, Lin. 1984. "Promise Her Everything: The Nuclear Power Industry's Agenda for Women." *Feminist Studies* 10 (2): 291–314.

Newman, R. 2001. "Making Environmental Politics: Women and Love Canal Activism." *Women's Studies Quarterly* 20 (1–2): 65–84.

Nihon Iraku Iryō Shien Nettowāku. 2014. *Fukushima Shiminhōshanō Sokuteijo Direkutori* [Directory of citizen radiation measuring organizations in Fukushima]. Tokyo: Nihon Iraku Iryo Shien Nettowāku.

Nitta Ikuko. 2012. "Hōshanō Kara Nigete" [Fleeing from radiation]. *Musubu* 492: 10–31.

"Nōsakubutsu kisechigoe tsugitsugi sanchi himei" [More and more food exceeds standards: Producers say standards too strict]. 2011. *Yomiuri Shinbun*, March 26.

"Nōsakubutsusyukkateishi, Gendankaide Kyūshokuni Eikyōnashi, Monkashō" [Stoppage of agricultural production, no impact now on school lunch, says minister of education]. 2011. *Nihon Keizai Shinbun*, March 22. http://www.nikkei.com/article/DGXNASDG22010_S1A320C1CC0000/.

Noshchenko, Andriy G., Oleksandra Y. Bondar, and Vira D. Drozdova. 2010. "Radiation-Induced Leukemia among Children Aged 0–5 Years at the Time of the Chernobyl Accident." *International Journal of Cancer* 127 (2): 412–26.

Nuclear Reform Monitoring Committee. n.d. "About the Nuclear Reform Monitoring Committee." http://www.nrmc.jp/en/about/index-e.html. Accessed September 24, 2014.

Ochi Koeda. 2014. "Kōjōsensukurīningude Kajōiryō Wa Attanoka" [Overdiagnosis in the screening for thyroid cancer?]. *Japan Business Press*, August 20. http://jbpress.ismedia.jp/articles/-/41510.

Odawara City Council. 2012. "Nōsanbutsuno Gakkōkyushokushiyōnikansuru Ketsugi" [Resolution on the use of produce in school lunches]. http://www.city.odawara.kanagawa.jp/global-image/units/96773/1-20120614145313.pdf.

Office of the Prime Minister. 2011. "Tokyodenryoku Ni Kansuru Keiei Zaimuchōsaiinkaihōkoku No Gaiyō" [Summary of report by the committee on TEPCO management and finance]. http://www.cas.go.jp/jp/seisaku/keieizaimutyousa/dai10/siryou2.pdf.

Ogawa Junko. 2013. "Soredemo Genshiryokuwo Suterarenaiwake" [The reason not to abandon nuclear energy]. *Eneco* 1: 26–30.

"Ogawa Junko." n.d. *Chou Chou*. http://www.win-japan.org/activity/pdf/others_ChuChu_ogawa.pdf. Accessed January 5, 2015.

"*Oishinbo* Hamonhirogaru" [*Oishinbo* impacts are spreading]. 2014.

"*Oishinbo* Hanadi Konkyoaru Senmonkara Hanronkaiken" [Experts commenting on *Oishinbo* problem, medical basis for nasal bleeding]. 2014. *Asahi Shinbun*, May 24.

"*Oishinbo* Hyōgen Ni Zannen, Kankyōshō Seimukan" [Regrettable, on *Oishinbo*, says Ministry of Environment's vice minister]. 2014. *Asahi Shinbun*, May 9.

Oisix Co. 2013. *Oisix Annual Report 2013*. Tokyo: Oisix Co. http://v4.eir-parts.net/v4Contents/View.aspx?cat=yuho_pdf&sid=1906304.

Okada, Hiroki. 2012. "An Anthropological Examination of Differences between the Great East Japan Earthquake and the Great Hanshin Earthquake." *Asian Anthropology* 11 (1): 55–63.

Okubo Chiwako. 2011. *Hōshanōni Makenai! Kantan Makurobiotikku Reshipi 88* [Don't succumb to radiation! Eighty-eight macrobiotic recipes]. Tokyo: Nosangyosonbuka Kyokai.

"Onajikondatede Bentō Fuannnuguenu Haha, Gyūnyū Kyohi Mo" [Concerned mothers prepare bento with the same menu, also rejecting milk]. 2012. *Tokyo Shinbun*, February 12.

Ong, Aihwa. 1996. "Cultural Citizenship as Subject-Making: Immigrants Negotiate Racial and Cultural Boundaries in the United States." *Current Anthropology* 37 (5): 737–62.

———. 2003. *Buddha Is Hiding: Refugees, Citizenship, the New America*. Berkeley: University of California Press.

———. 2006. *Neoliberalism as Exception: Mutations in Citizenship and Sovereignty*. Durham, NC: Duke University Press.

Onuma Junichi. 2013. "Shokuhinnadono Hōshanō Sokuteitaisei No Bappontekina Kaikaku Ni Tsuite" [Fundamental reform of the system of monitoring radioactive materials in food]. Tokyo: Genshiryokushimin Iinkai [Citizens' Commission on Nuclear Energy]. http://www.ccnejapan.com/archive/2013/.

Onuma Yasushi. 2012. *Sekai Ga Mita Fukushimagenpatsu Saigai 3* [Fukushima nuclear disaster through the world's eye 3]. Tokyo: Ryokufu Shuppan.

Osaka High Court. 2008. *Decision of the Osaka High Court on the Atomic Bomb-Caused Injuries Certification Case.* www.courts.go.jp/app/files/hanrei_jp/731/036731_hanrei.pdf.

Papadopoulos, Dimitris. 2011. "Alter-Ontologies: Towards a Constituent Politics in Technoscience." *Social Studies of Science* 41 (2): 177–201.

Papadopoulos, Dimitris, Niamh Stephenson, and Vassilis Tsianos. 2008. *Escape Routes: Control and Subversion in the Twenty-First Century.* London: Pluto Press.

Pekkanen, R. 2006. *Japan's Dual Civil Society: Members without Advocates.* Palo Alto, CA: Stanford University Press.

Pellizzoni, L., and M. Ylönen. 2012. *Neoliberalism and Technoscience: Critical Assessments.* Burlington, VT: Ashgate.

Petryna, Adriana. 2002. *Life Exposed: Biological Citizens after Chernobyl.* Princeton, NJ: Princeton University Press.

Pew Research Center. 2014. "Population Change in the U.S. and the World from 1950 to 2050." January 30. http://www.pewglobal.org/2014/01/30/chapter-4-population-change-in-the-u-s-and-the-world-from-1950-to-2050/.

Pharr, Susan J. 2003. "Targeting by an Activist State: Japan as a Civil Society Model." In *The State of Civil Society in Japan*, edited by Susan J. Pharr and Frank J. Schwartz, 316–36. Cambridge: Cambridge University Press.

Physicians for Social Responsibility, et al. 2013. "Annotated Critique of United Nations Scientific Committee on the Effects of Atomic Radiation (UNSCEAR) October 2013 Fukushima Report to the UN General Assembly." International Physicians for the Prevention of Nuclear War, October 18. http://www.ippnw.de/commonFiles/pdfs/Atomenergie/Ausfuehrlicher_Kommentar_zum_UNSCEAR_Fukushima_Bericht_2013__Englisch_.pdf.

Proctor, R., and L. Schiebinger. 2008. *Agnotology: The Making and Unmaking of Ignorance.* Palo Alto, CA: Stanford University Press.

"Prof. Nagayama of Kyusyu University Proposes Food Standards." 2012. *Nishi Nihon Shinbun*, January 18.

Public Security Intelligence Agency. 2006. "Naigaijōsei No Kaikototenbō 2006" [Review and prospects of domestic and international situations 2006]. http://www.moj.go.jp/psia/kouan_naigai_naigai18_naigai18-04.html.

———. 2012. "Naigaijōsei No Kaikototenbō 2012" [Review and prospects of domestic and international situations 2012]. http://www.moj.go.jp/content/000084409.pdf.

"Purometeusu no Wana Ishi Zensen e" [Prometheus trap, doctors on the front line]. 2013. *Asahi Shinbun*, November 6.

Radiation Council. 2012. "Minutes of the 126th Meeting of the Radiation Council." Ministry of Education, Culture, Sports, Science and Technology. http://labor-manabiya.news.coocan.jp/shiryoushitsu/shokuhin_shinkijyun/houshasenshingikai_126_gijiroku.pdf.

Radiation Effects Research Foundation. 2012. "RERF's Views on Residual Radiation." December 8. http://www.rerf.jp/news/pdf/residualrad_ps_e.pdf.

Ramos-Zayas, Ana Y. 2012. *Street Therapists: Race, Affect, and Neoliberal Personhood in Latino Newark*. Chicago: University of Chicago Press.

Rancière, Jacques. 1998. *Disagreement: Politics and Philosophy*. Minneapolis: University of Minnesota Press.

———. 2003. "Politics and Aesthetics, Interview with Peter Hallward." *Angelaki* 8 (2): 191–212.

Reconstruction Agency. 2014. "Hōshasen Ni Tsuiteno Tadashii Chishikiwo" [Have correct knowledge of radiation]. http://dwl.gov-online.go.jp/video/cao/dl/public_html/gov/pdf/paper/kijishita/ph624b.pdf.

Rose, Nikolas. 1993. "Government, Authority and Expertise in Advanced Liberalism." *Economy and Society* 22 (3): 283–99.

Rottenberg, Catherine. 2014. "The Rise of Neoliberal Feminism." *Cultural Studies* 28 (3): 418–37.

Rowe, G., and L. Flewer. 2005. "A Typology of Public Engagement Mechanisms: Science." *Science, Technology, and Human Values* 30 (2): 251–90.

Saito Hiroshi. 2010. "Monsutā Pearento No Taiōsaku Ni Kansuru Paradaimu Henkan" [Paradigm shift in responses to monster parents]. *Bukkyodaigaku Kyoikugakubugakkaikiyo* 9: 111–22.

Sakakibara Takahito. 2014. "'Hōshasen No Anshin' Hontō? Gan to Genpatsujiko No Kankei Wa" [Is it true that "we don't need to worry about radiation"? Relationships between cancer and the nuclear accident]. *Chunichi Shinbun*, April 8. http://iryou.chunichi.co.jp/article/detail/20140409161307207.

Samuels, Richard J. 2013a. *3.11: Disaster and Change in Japan*. Ithaca, NY: Cornell University Press.

———. 2013b. "Japan's Rhetoric of Crisis: Prospects for Change after 3.11." *Journal of Japanese Studies* 39 (1): 97–120.

Sanami Yuko. 2013. *Joshi to Aikoku* [Joshi and patriotism]. Tokyo: Shodensha.

Sandberg, Sheryl. 2013. *Lean In: Women, Work, and the Will to Lead*. New York: Knopf.

Sand, Jordan. 2012. "Living with Uncertainty after March 11, 2011." *Journal of Asian Studies* 71 (2): 313–18.

Satō Hiroaki, and Koyuki Yamane. 2012. "Hōshaseibusshitsu Fukenshutsu No Yami" [Doubt on "radiation not detected"]. *Nikkei Business Magazine*, September 3: 10–12.

Satō Kazunori. 2011. "Gyōmuyōjuyōnitaiōshita Yasaisanchi No Hanbaisenrya-kuto Soshikitaisei" [Cooperative marketing and organization in vegetable-producing areas adjusting for business use]. *Fūdosisutemu Kenkyū* 18 (1): 41–45.

Satō Ukiya. 2005. "Gakkūkyūshokuno Kenkyū" [Research on school lunches]. *Iwate Daigaku Kenkyu Nenpo.*

Schiebinger, L. 2007. *Plants and Empire: Colonial Bioprospecting in the Atlantic World.* Cambridge, MA: Harvard University Press.

Schreurs, Miranda M. 2013. "The International Reaction to the Fukushima Nuclear Accident and Implications for Japan." In *Fukushima: A Political Economic Analysis of a Nuclear Disaster,* edited by Miranda M. Schreurs and Fumikazu Yoshida, 1–16. Sapporo: Hokkaido University Press.

Sclove, R. E. 2000. "Town Meetings on Technology: Consensus Conference as Democratic Participation." In *Science, Technology and Democracy,* edited by D. Lee Kleinman, 33–48. Albany: State University of New York Press.

Scott, James C. 1990. *Domination and the Arts of Resistance: Hidden Transcripts.* New Haven, CT: Yale University Press.

———. 2008. *Weapons of the Weak: Everyday Forms of Peasant Resistance.* New Haven, CT: Yale University Press.

Seager, Joni. 1996. "Hysterical Housewives and Other Mad Women." In *Feminist Political Ecology: Global Issues and Local Experiences,* edited by Dianne E. Rocheleau, Barbara Thomas-Slayter, and Esther Wangari, 271–83. New York: Routledge.

"Seifu Genpatsu Baisyōde Tōden Ni Tsuikashien, Sōgakugochōen" [Additional government help to TEPCO for compensation, exceeding 5 trillion yen]. 2014. *Yomiuri Shinbun,* August 8.

Sekine Shinichi. 2013. "Kyūshokuni Fukushimamai" [Fukushima rice in the school lunch program]. *Asahi Shinbun,* October 5.

Sekiya Naoya. 2003. "Fūhyōhigai No Shakaishinri" [Social psychology of Fūhyōhigai]. *Saigaijōhō,* no. 1: 78–89.

———. 2011. *Fūhyōhigai* [Harmful rumors]. Tokyo: Kobunsha.

Seko Hiroko. 2012. "Hisaichishokuhinwo Kau? Kawanai? Ankētochōosano Kek-kakara" [Buying or not buying food from affected areas: Results from a survey]. *Food Communication Compass,* March 8. http://www.foocom.net/column/answer/5927/.

"Shichōni Kōkaishitumonjō." February 2012. http://www.ustream.tv/recorded/29595828. Accessed March 4, 2014.

Shimizu Nanako. 2013. "Genshiryokusaigainiyoru Hisaishashiensesakupakkēji Ni Kansuru Saiyōbōsho Teishutsuno Hōkoku" [Report on resubmission of demands regarding victims' assistance package]. http://cmps.utsunomiya-u.ac.jp/fsp/fsp20130409.pdf.

Shirabe Masashi. 2013. "Ubawareru Riariti: Teisenryōhibau Wo Meguru Kagaku/ kagaku No Tsukawarekata" [Deprived of reality: Science and the use of science on low-dose exposure]. In *Posuto 3.11 No Kagaku to Seiji* [Science and politics after the disaster of March 11 in Japan], 51–82. Kyoto: Nakanishiya.

"Shokuhin No Hōshaseibusshitsukijyun Hijyō Ni Gimon" [Questioning the radiation standards for food]. 2014. *Independent Web Journal*, March 5. http://iwj.co .jp/wj/open/archives/127855.

"Shokuhin No Hōshaseibusshitsukijyun Kanwa Kentō" [Will explore easing radiation standards for food]. 2014. *47 News*, March 5. http://www.47news.jp /CN/201403/CN2014030501002264.html.

Shrader-Frechette, Kristin, and Lars Persson. 2002. "Ethical, Logical and Scientific Problems with the New ICRP Proposals." *Journal of Radiological Protection* 22 (2): 149–61.

Shufuno Tomo, ed. 2011. *Hōshanō No Dokudashi! Genmai, Miso Kaisō Reshipi Nihon No Shokuno Chikara* [Detoxing radiation: The power of Japanese food: Brown rice, miso and seaweed recipes]. Tokyo: Shufuno Tomosha.

"Shutoken Supesharu" [Metropolitan area special]. 2011. NHK, September. http:// www.nhk.or.jp/shutoken/special/opinion/opinion110930_04.html.

Slater, David. 2014. "Fukushima Women against Nuclear Power: Finding a Voice from Tohoku." *Asia-Pacific Journal Japan Focus* 117 (November 11). http://www .japanfocus.org/events/view/117.

Slater, David H., Rika Morioka, and Haruka Danzuka. 2014. "Micro-Politics of Radiation." *Critical Asian Studies* 46 (3): 485–508.

Slovic, Paul. 1999. "Trust, Emotion, Sex, Politics, and Science: Surveying the Risk-Assessment Battlefield." *Risk Analysis* 19 (4): 689–701.

Soh, C. Sarah. 2008. *The Comfort Women: Sexual Violence and Postcolonial Memory in Korea and Japan*. Chicago: University of Chicago Press.

Star, Susan L. 1999. "The Ethnography of Infrastructure." *American Behavioral Scientist* 43 (3): 377–91.

Steinhoff, Patricia. 2007. "Radical Outcasts versus Three Kinds of Police: Constructing Limits in Japanese Anti-Emperor Protests." In *New Perspectives in Political Ethnography*, edited by Lauren Joseph, Matthew Mahler, and Javier Auyero, 60–87. New York: Springer.

Sternsdorff-Cisterna, Nicolas. 2015. "Food after Fukushima: Risk and Scientific Citizenship in Japan." *American Anthropologist* 117: 455–67.

Suga Hidemi. 2012. *Hangenpatsu No Shisōshi* [Ideological history of antinuclear movement]. Tokyo: Chikuma Shobo.

Sugiman, Toshio. 2014. "Lessons Learned from the 2011 Debacle of the Fukushima Nuclear Power Plant." *Public Understanding of Science* 23 (3): 254–67.

Sumner, David. 2007. "Health Effects Resulting from the Chernobyl Accident." *Medicine, Conflict and Survival* 23 (1): 31–45.

Suzuki Shinichi. 2014. "Fukushimaken Deno Kōjōsengan Kensakekkano Genjyō" [On the results of thyroid cancer screening in Fukushima Prefecture]. Interview. TEPCO Fukushiam No. 1 Nuclear Accident, May 26. http://www.jaero .or.jp/data/02topic/fukushima/interview/suzuki_t.html.

Swyngedouw, Erik. 2010. "Apocalypse Forever? Post-Political Populism and the Spectre of Climate Change." Theory, Culture and Society 27 (2–3): 213–32.

Tabuchi, Hiroko. 2014. "Reversing Course, Japan Makes Push to Restart Dormant Nuclear Plants." New York Times, February 26.

Tajima Emi. 1999. Ekorojī Undō to Jendāteki Shiten [Ecology movement and gender perspectives]. 30. Tokyo: Gakuyo Shobo.

Takahashi Hiroko. 2012. Fūin Sareta Hiroshima Nagasaki [Classified Hiroshima and Nagasaki]. Tokyo: Gaifusha.

Takahashi Kuniko. 2012. "Shokuhin No Hōshasenosen to Fūdo Fadizumu" [Radiation contamination of food and food faddism]. Wedge, February. http://wedge .ismedia.jp/articles/-/1684?page=2.

Takatori Atsushi. 2014. "Seifukōhō Hōshasen Nitsuiteno Tadashii Chishikiwo No Mondai" [The problem with the government PR: "Have correct knowledge of radiation"]. E-Wave, August 19. http://www.eritokyo.jp/independent/takatori-fnp0043.htm.

Takayanagi Nagatada. 2006. Fūdo Shisutemu No Kūkan Kōzōron [Global transformation of special structure in agrofood systems]. Tokyo: Tsukuba Shobo.

Takeya Miso Co. n.d. "Miso Niyotte Genbakukōishōga Sukunakute Sunda" [Thanks to miso, radiation exposure effect was mitigated]. Miso Health Report. http:// www.takeya-miso.co.jp/column/008.html. Accessed May 15, 2014.

Tanaka, Yutaka. 2007. "Japanese Attitudes toward Genetically Modified (GM) Foods from JGSS-2005 Data." JGSS Research Series 3: 95–106.

Taussig, Michael T. 1999. Defacement: Public Secrecy and the Labor of the Negative. Palo Alto, CA: Stanford University Press.

Terashima Hideya. 2014. "Nogyōfukkōtojyōno Minamisomashi Wo Osotta Genpatsufunjinmondaieno Ikari" [Angered by nuclear power plant debris contamination, Minamisoma City struggles to rebuild its agriculture]. Blogos.com, August 6. http://blogos.com/article/91930/.

Tiberghien, Yves. 2014. "Thirty Years of Neo-Liberal Reforms in Japan." In The Great Transformation of Japanese Capitalism, edited by Sébastien Lechevalier, 26–55. London: Routledge.

Tierney, Kathleen, and Christine Bevc. 2010. "Disaster as War: Militarism and the Social Construction of Disaster in New Orleans." In The Sociology of Katrina: Perspectives on a Modern Catastrophe, edited by David L. Brunsma, David Overfelt, and Steven Picou, 35–50. Lanham, MD: Rowman and Littlefield.

"Tōden Genpatsu No Sōchikoshōwo Inpei" [TEPCO hid nuclear power plant accidents]. 2007. Nikkei BP Net, February 1. http://www.nikkeibp.co.jp/news /biz07q1/524352/.

Tōhoku Electricity Power Company. 2014. "Kawaiiga Sekaiwo Kaeru Wakai Josei Dakara Dekirukoto" [Transforming the world by Kawaii: Only young women can do it]. February. http://www.tohoku-epco.co.jp/fukyu/report/contents /f47_joshinokurashi/index.html.

Tokuda Hiroto. 2003. "Shokuhinanzenkihonhō Oyobi Kaiseishokuhineiseihō No Hihanteki Kentō" [Critical analysis of food safety basic law and amended food sanitation act]. *Ryudaihogaku*, no. 70: 1–26.

Topçu, Sezin. 2013. "Chernobyl Empowerment? Exporting 'Participatory Governance' to Contaminated Territories." In *Toxicants, Health and Regulation since 1945*, edited by Soraya Boudia and Nathalie Jas, 135–58. London: Pickering & Chatto.

Trivedi, Akhilesh, and Mohammed A. Hannan. 2004. "Radiation and Cardiovascular Diseases." *Journal of Environmental Pathology, Toxicology and Oncology* 23 (2). http://www.dl.begellhouse.com/journals/0ff459a57a4c08d0,69988c136ea15 9a9,2a0a3be732d18aa4.html.

Tsutsui, Takako, Naoko Muramatsu, and Sadanori Higashino. 2013. "Changes in Perceived Filial Obligation Norms among Coresident Family Caregivers in Japan." *Gerontologist*, September. http://gerontologist.oxfordjournals.org/content/early /2013/09/04/geront.gnt093.

Tuana, Nancy. 2006. "The Speculum of Ignorance: The Women's Health Movement and Epistemologies of Ignorance." *Hypatia* 21 (3): 1–19.

UNSCEAR. 2012. "The Chernobyl Accident: UNSCEAR's Assessments of the Radiation Effects." July 16. http://www.unscear.org/unscear/en/chernobyl .html#Summary.

Valaskivi, Katja. 2013. "A Brand New Future? Cool Japan and the Social Imaginary of the Branded Nation." *Japan Forum* 25: 485–504. http://www.tandfonline .com/doi/abs/10.1080/09555803.2012.756538.

Wacquant, Loïc. 2010. "Crafting the Neoliberal State: Workfare, Prisonfare, and Social Insecurity." *Sociological Forum* 25: 197–220.

Wakakuwa, Midori, and Kumiko Fujimura-Fanselow. 2011. "Backlash against Gender Inequality after 2000." In *Transforming Japan: How Feminism and Diversity Are Making a Difference*, 337–59. New York: Feminist Press at CUNY.

Wakamatsu Jōtaro. 2012. *Fukushimakakusaikimin* [Abandoned people: Fukushima nuclear disaster]. Tokyo: Coal-Sack.

Walker, Brett L. 2009. *Toxic Archipelago: A History of Industrial Disease in Japan*. Seattle: University of Washington Press.

Watanabe Mikiko. 2004. "Multilateral Approach to the Realities of the Chernobyl NPP Accident: Summing up the Consequences of the Accident Twenty Years After." Kyoto University Research Reactor Institute. http://www.rri.kyoto-u .ac.jp/PUB/report/04_kr/133.html.

Watanuki Reiko, ed. 1987. *Hairo Ni Mukete: Josei Ni Totte Genpatsu Towa Nanika* [Toward decommissioning nuclear reactors]. Tokyo: Hinhyoron.

Weigt, Jill. 2006. "Compromises to Carework: The Social Organization of Mothers' Experiences in the Low-Wage Labor Market after Welfare Reform." *Social Problems* 53 (3): 332–51.

Welsh, Ian, and Brian Wynne. 2013. "Science, Scientism and Imaginaries of Publics in the UK: Passive Objects, Incipient Threats." *Science as Culture* 22 (4): 540–66.

Wilkening, Kenneth E. 2004. *Acid Rain Science and Politics in Japan: A History of Knowledge and Action toward Sustainability.* Cambridge, MA: MIT Press.

Windfuhr, M., and J. Jonsén. 2005. *Food Sovereignty: Towards Democracy in Localized Food Systems.* London: Intermediate Technology.

Wolch, Jennifer R. 1990. *The Shadow State: Government and Voluntary Sector in Transition.* New York: Foundation Center.

Women in Nuclear. 2011. "19th WiN Global Annual Conference Fukushima Declaration." http://www.win-japan.org/activity/pdf/Fukushima_Declaration.pdf.

Women in Nuclear Global. 2015. "What We Do." Accessed October 26. http://win-global.org/about/what.

Woolgar, Steve, and Javier Lezaun, eds. 2013a. "Special Issue: A Turn to Ontology in Science and Technology Studies?" *Social Studies of Science* 43 (3).

———. 2013b. "The Wrong Bin Bag: A Turn to Ontology in Science and Technology Studies?" *Social Studies of Science* 43 (3): 321–40.

World Economic Forum. 2014. "Global Gender Gap Index." http://reports.weforum.org/global-gender-gap-report-2014/rankings/. Accessed May 2, 2015.

World Nuclear Association. 2014. "Nuclear Power Plants and Earthquakes." May. http://www.world-nuclear.org/info/Safety-and-Security/Safety-of-Plants/Nuclear-Power-Plants-and-Earthquakes/.

Wynne, B. 1992. "Misunderstood Misunderstanding: Social Identities and Public Uptake of Science." *Public Understanding of Science* 1 (3): 281–304.

Yagi Ekou. 2007. "Daigakuinkyōyōkyōikutoshiteno Kagakugijyutsukomyunikēshon Kyōikuno Teian" [A proposal for science communication education in liberal arts in graduate school]. *Communication Design,* 121–46.

Yamaguchi, Tomomi. 2014. "'Gender Free' Feminism in Japan: A Story of Mainstreaming and Backlash." *Feminist Studies* 40 (3): 541–72.

Yamazaki Yukiko. 2008. *Monsutā Pearento No Shōtai* [Reality of monster parents]. Tokyo: Chuohokishuppan.

Yamazoe Yasushi. 2011. "Ronten Ni Kansuru Zachō Memo" [Memo by the chair on key issues]. Food Safety Commission. https://www.fsc.go.jp/fsciis/meetingMaterial/show/kai20110726so1.

Yoshioka Masahiko. 2014. "Shinsaigo No Fukushima Ken No Jinkōhenka" [Demographic change in Fukushima after the disasters]. Fukushima Jichi Kensyu Senta. http://www.f-jichiken.or.jp/column/160/yosioka160.html.

Yoshizawa Yumiko. 2011. "Hayashi Shichō Intabyū No Nakade Tokuni Kininaru Kyūshokuno Hōshasen Sokutei" [Particularly interesting interview with Mayor Hayashi: Measuring radiation in school lunches]. *Hamarepo*, November. http://hamarepo.com/story.php?story_id=615.

Young, Iris Marion. 2000. *Inclusion and Democracy*. Oxford: Oxford University Press.

Zensho Co. n.d. "Food Safety FAQs." http://www.zensho.co.jp/jp/safety/faq/.

INDEX

Note: f = figure; m = map; t = table

Abe Shinzo, 22–23, 33, 137, 141–43
academic pedigree society (*gakureki shakai*), 101
acid rain, 160n12
activism: antinuclear, 19–20, 68, 80, 92–94, 111–13, 116–18, 168nn4–5; antiwar, 169n6; and citizen science, 2, 4, 7, 20, 105–8, 111–13, 122, 128–31; contamination, 6–7, 17–19, 35, 81–94, 105–6, 119; CRMOs and nonactivism, 2, 4, 104–7, 120–21, 128, 156; environmental, 20, 35, 113, 119; feminist, 5, 21, 71; gendered constraints on, 17–19, 21, 24–25, 35, 79–80, 94–96, 133–34, 149–50, 167n14, 167nn16–17; and motherhood, 24–25, 79–80, 90–94, 97–98; and New Left politics, 117–20, 168nn4–5; and neoliberalism, 3, 5–7, 17–19, 107, 120–22, 133–34. *See also* CRMOs; safe school lunch movement
activist joshi, 79–80, 94–98, 102, 167nn14–17. *See also* postfeminist gender settlement; safe school lunch movement
activist mothering, 92. *See also* motherhood; safe school lunch movement
Aegerter, Irene, 69–70, 165n11
Aeon supermarkets, 47–48, 163n17

Aera (magazine), 46
Agamben, Giorgio, 145
aging of nuclear reactors, 111–12, 140, 154
aging of population, 23, 83, 150, 152–53
agriculture, 22, 31–32, 82, 98, 141–45; and consumer avoidance, 7, 31–32, 84–85, 100; and contamination, 7–9, 99, 141–42, 159n5; smart, 143–45, 170n4. *See also* farming
Akashi Makoto, 42
Aldrich, Daniel, 14
Allison, Anne, 152
All Japan Parents Who Want Safe School Lunch, 90
Amano Yukiya, 43
anshin (peace of mind), 53, 139
anticipation, regime of, 133–34, 142–45
antifeminism, 21–22, 71, 81
antinuclear movement, 19–20, 68, 80, 92–94, 111–13, 116–18, 168nn4–5
aquaponics, 144, 170n4
aspirationalism, neoliberal, 11, 13, 25–26, 57, 71–73, 142–43, 151
Association for Future's Creation of Tamura and Children (AFTC), 64–65
Association of Women for Postnuclear, 80

Association pour le Contrôle de la Radio-
activité de l'Ouest (ACRO), 112
Association to Protect Children from
Radiation, 94, 113
Association to Think about Aging
Nuclear Reactors in Fukushima
(Fukushima Rōkyugenpatsu wo
Kangaerukai), 112
atmospheric testing of nuclear bombs,
89, 93, 112, 162n14
Atomic Bomb Casualty Commission
(ABCC), 39, 40, 162n12
atomic bomb survivors (hibakusha),
38–40, 145, 162n12
Azuma Hirokatsu, 50

bare life, 145–47, 150
bari-kyari (career-oriented woman), 7
Bayat, Asef, 156
Beck, Ulrich, 55
becquereled (bekureta/bekurenai),
126–27
becquerel-free food, 46–48, 50–53, 94
beef. See cesium beef scandal
Belarus, 29–30, 102
Bikini Atoll, 93
Borovoy, Amy, 97
bovine spongiform encephalopathy (mad
cow disease), 13, 32, 58
breast cancer, 96
breast milk, 47, 111
Brown, Mark, 130
Brown, Phil, 159n2
Brown, Wendy, 121–22
bubble economy, 22, 71, 83
bullying, 36, 91, 166n6

cadmium, 19, 160
cancer, 40–43, 63, 96, 146, 153
care work, 16, 18–19, 25, 132–33, 149–50,
153, 161n9, 171n6
cesium: in the body, 41–42; in the
environment, 8, 36, 99, 135, 140, 162n10;
in food, 50, 59, 84, 115, 127–28, 162n10,
163nn17–19, 166n5, 170n3; measurement, 14, 89, 104, 126–27, 109, 139–40;

standards, 30, 31t, 108, 161n3. See also
CRMOs; specific foods
cesium beef scandal, 32, 47–48, 78–79,
84–86, 88, 163nn17–18, 165n4, 170n3
Chernobyl nuclear accident, 14, 66, 68,
102, 145–46, 154, 164; ETHOS, 61–64;
health impacts, 40; Japanese reaction,
82, 86, 93, 107–8, 135, 148–49; safety
standards, 30, 161n3
Chhem, Rethy, 42
Chiba Prefecture, 3m, 8
chisan-chishō (local food), 27, 31, 53, 98,
141, 166n6, 168n21
Chisso Chemical Corporation, 119, 160n11
Chūkaku-ha, 118–19
citizen radiation-measuring organizations. See CRMOs
Citizen Radiation-Measuring Stations
network, 109, 134
citizen science (shiminkagakusha), 20,
159n2; and CRMOs, 2, 4, 14, 25, 105–7,
122–24, 128–31, 133–34, 156–58; and
neoliberal citizenship, 4–7, 15–17,
106–7, 120–25, 128–31, 134, 154–56; and
politics, 2, 4–7, 14–17, 25, 81, 105–6, 117,
148, 155–58, 160n9; and women, 5–7,
17–19, 21, 24–26, 81, 133–34. See also
CRMOs; safe school lunch movement
Citizen Science (Irwin), 159n2
Citizen's Nuclear Information Center, 20,
108
citizen-subject. See neoliberal citizen-
subject
civil society, 10, 14–17, 106, 121, 136, 151,
171n1
claimer parents (kurēmā), 87
class stratification, 18, 24, 52–54, 57, 73,
76, 82
Cold War, 2, 82
Commission de Recherche et d'Information Indépendantes sur la Radioactivité
(CRIIRAD), 108–9
communication, risk, 21, 24, 52, 55–66,
64–72, 76–77, 164nn3–6, 164n9
communication, women-to-women, 21,
24, 56–58, 68–76

communism, 19–20, 118–19, 168n5, 169n6

Consumer Affairs Agency, 59–60, 164n4

consumer avoidance, 7, 27–28, 30–34, 36, 38, 51, 56, 60, 161n5

consumer cooperatives, 27, 30, 108, 113

consumerism, 58, 95–97

consumer rights, 38, 113

contamination: decline over time, 9, 99, 132, 136, 141; gendered concern about, 17, 34–35, 161n9; social construction of, 1, 6, 11, 13, 24–26, 133–34, 136–37, 141–45, 157–58; temporal politics of, 133, 136–37, 141–45. *See also* activism; citizen science; CRMOs; food policing; food radiation testing; external radiation; internal radiation; pollution; radiation; safe school lunch movement; safety standards

contamination, environmental, 13, 45–48, 62–63, 65–66, 99, 105–7, 140–42, 146, 162n10. *See also* cesium; citizen science; decontamination; external radiation; pollution; safety standards

contamination, food, 1–2, 7–10, 29–32, 49–52, 69, 78–79, 84, 103, 136–38. *See also* cesium; CRMOs; food policing; food radiation testing; food safety scandals; internal radiation; safe school lunch movement; safety standards

contamination activism, 6–7, 17–19, 35, 81–94, 105–6, 119

contamination measurement as means to make the invisible visible, 4, 14, 89, 115, 124, 128. *See also* CRMOs; food radiation testing; safety standards

cost-benefit calculation of protection, 62–63, 66–67

CRMOS, 1, 4, 14, 17, 25; affective role, 128, 138–39; and antinuclear politics, 2, 108, 111–12, 115–18, 128, 134; after Chernobyl accident, 107–8, 135; declining numbers, 132–36, 141; and disaster preparedness, 140–41, 154; findings of contamination, 109, 111, 114–15, 126–28; founders' backgrounds, 113–16; and government

testing services, 108, 110–11, 126, 135–39, 141, 157, 168n3, 170n1; information exchange function, 125–26, 134, 137–40; locations, 108–9, 110m; networks, 108–9, 134, 140; and nonactivism, 2, 4, 104–7, 116–20, 122, 128, 156; and scientism, 129, 131–32, 156–57; testing as neutral act, 105, 117, 122–24; testing as political act, 123–31, 147; training, 108–9, 139–40, 169n8, 170n3; watchdog function, 109, 111, 114–15, 126, 137–38. *See also* citizen science

data sharing, 13, 125–26, 134, 140

Dean, Mitchell, 10

decontamination: bodily, 48–51; environmental, 36, 99, 162n10

decontamination cost, 46–47, 62–63

democracy, 9, 14–15, 101–2, 130, 146, 151, 160n9

Democratic Party, 23, 80

depoliticization, 4, 19, 25, 96, 122, 124, 143, 157

detoxification, 48–49

disaster capitalism, 24, 46–53

disaster preparedness, 134, 140–41, 143, 150, 154

disaster prevention, 134, 143, 154

disaster recovery, 10, 38, 46–47, 64, 136–37, 141–44, 170n4

disaster studies, 120, 144

Dolhinow, Rebecca, 18, 121–22, 150

Eat to Support campaign, 7, 8, 10

ecofeminism, 160n10, 161n9

ecological modernization, 19, 160n10, 160n12

economic effects of Fukushima accident, 32, 46–47, 62–63. *See also* food producers; fūhyōhigai

education: and gender, 11, 21, 71, 101; science and technology, 164n5; and shokuiku (food education) campaign, 37, 82, 98, 166n6

Eliasoph, Nina, 171n1

mercury, 19, 160
Merton, Robert, 160n9
Migakiichigo ("shining strawberries") brand, 142–44, 170n4
milk: contaminated, 2, 29, 45, 55, 94, 127; safety standards for, 30, 31t; in school lunch, 82–83, 165n3, 166n6
milk, breast, 47, 111
miso, 48–49
Mitsui Corporation, 134, 160n11
Mitsui Environmental Fund, 134
Miyagi Prefecture, 31, 115–16, 142, 170n4
monster parents (*monsutā pearento*), 87, 166
Moodie, Megan, 18
Mori Masako, 56
Morris-Suzuki, Tessa, 148, 152, 156, 159n6
Mother's Congress, 93
mother's food (*ofukuro no aji*), 37
Mothers' Group to Investigate Early Radiation Exposure, 91–92
motherhood, 22–25, 28, 37, 53–54, 71, 79–81, 85, 90–94, 97–98, 101. *See also* joshi power; safe school lunch movement
Murphy, Michelle, 5, 125
mushrooms, 84, 89, 111, 126–127, 148, 166n5, 166n9, 170n1

Nagasaki, 3m, 38–39, 145
Nagayama Junya, 30
Nakagawa Keiichi, 42
Nakagawa Yasuo, 162n14
Naples, Nancy, 92
nationalism, postdisaster, 38, 120, 143, 145, 147, 151
National Public Security Intelligence Agency, 118, 169n6
NAZEN (Subeteno Genpatsu Imasugu Nakusō! Zenkoku Kaigi) (Let's Abolish All Nuclear Reactors Right Now!), 118
Nelson, Lin, 57, 163n1
neoliberal citizen-subject, 5, 11–13, 15–17, 56, 67, 127, 151, 155–56. *See also* citizen science: neoliberal citizenship; neoliber-

alism; postfeminism; postfeminist gender settlement
neoliberalism, 5, 10–12, 15–16, 121; anticipatory regime of, 133–34, 142–45; and avoidance of politics, 107, 120–23, 129, 131, 151; and emotion, 76, 142, 155, 157; and social protection, 12, 18–19, 83, 132–33, 151–52, 154, 165n2, 171n1, 171n6
New Standards for Radioactive Materials in Food (video), 42
NGO-ization, 16, 103, 121, 171n1
Nitta Ikuko, 52–53
Niwa Otsura, 64
Noda Yoshihiko, 137
nō-mama (radiation brain moms), 24, 27–29, 35, 38, 44, 46
nonprofit organization structure, 136
nuclear energy, 57, 60–62, 66, 68–71, 75–77, 92–94, 140; and feminism, 69, 163n1; opposition to, 2, 19–20, 68, 80, 92–94, 111–13, 116–18, 168nn4–5; sustainability of, 19; women's perspective on, 21, 24, 56–58, 68–70, 72–76, 164n10
nuclear industry, 24, 47, 60–62, 102, 125, 138, 140, 162n14, 164n8; as male-dominated field, 69, 72–73, 164n10. *See also* nuclear energy; nuclear village; risk communication; United States: nuclear industry; utility industry
Nuclear Information and Resource Service, 112
nuclear organizations, international, 40–41, 43, 61–67, 162nn12–14, 164n10
nuclear reactors, 19, 32, 111–12, 115, 140, 154, 160n13, 170n2. *See also* Chernobyl nuclear accident; Fukushima Daiichi (No. 1) Nuclear Power Plant; Fukushima nuclear accident
Nuclear Reform Monitoring Committee (TEPCO), 72
Nuclear Safety Commission, 30, 161
nuclear village (*genshiryokumura*), 2, 21, 43–44, 68–70, 80, 97, 123